Ketoger Vegetarian

This Book Includes 3 Manuscripts:

Vegan Ketogenic: The Best Kept Secret for Amazing Health & Easy Fat Loss

Carb Cycling: The Simple Way to Work With Your Body to Burn Fat & Build Muscle

DASH Diet: Overcome Hypertension, Lose Weight,

and Experience a New Level of Health

Vegan Ketogenic Diet

The Best Kept Secret for Amazing Health & Easy Fat Loss

Thomas Rohmer

Copyright © 2018
Rohmerfitness All rights reserved.

No part of this publication may be reproduced, distributed, or
transmitted in any form or by any means, including photocopying, recording, or other electronic or mechanical methods, without the prior written permission and consent of the publisher, except in the in the case of brief quotations embodied in product reviews and certain other non-commercial uses permitted by copyright law.

Disclaimer:

This guide has been created for informational and reference purposes only. The author, publisher, and any other affiliated parties cannot be held in any way accountable for any personal injuries or damage allegedly resulting from the information contained herein, or from any misuse of such guidance. Although strict measures have been taken to provide accurate information, the parties involved with the creation and publication of this guide take no responsibility for any issues that many arise from alleged discrepancies contained herein. It is strongly recommended that you consult a physician, personal trainer, and nutritionist prior to commencing this or any other workout or diet plan. This guide is not a substitute for professional personal guidance from a qualified medical professional. If you feel pain or discomfort at any point during exercises contained herein, cease the activity immediately and seek medical guidance.

Before You Begin:

Get the Latest Scoop on the Most Cutting Edge Info on Health & Fitness!

As thanks for picking up this book, I'd love to offer you the chance to maximize your results by getting exclusive info on health and fitness.

You'll be the first to know when I publish new books, and you'll receive exclusive content on health and fitness that I only share with people on my list.

Simply click the link directly below and get started on the path to the healthiest version of yourself today!

https://rohmerfitness.lpages.co/kindle-sign-up/

Table of Contents

Chapter 1: It's Time to Take Back Control of Our Health.....................9
Chapter 2: What is the Ketogenic Diet..........11
Chapter 3: Health Benefits of the Ketogenic Diet...........16
Chapter 4: What is a Vegan Lifestyle?..........19
Chapter 5: Health Benefits of a Vegan Diet.23
Chapter 6: Why Combine a Vegan and Ketogenic Diet?.............32
Chapter 7: Setting Up Your Vegan Ketogenic Diet.............35
Chapter 8: What to Do for Exercise.............46
Chapter 9: 53 Vegan and Ketogenic Recipes...................51
Chapter 10: Frequently Asked Questions...117

Introduction:

Getting and staying healthy is definitely something that Americans are challenged with today. Two-thirds of the American population are either overweight or obese (1), and over half a million Americans die each year due to cardiovascular disease (2). Not all of it is completely our fault though. Many of the diets that exist today simply set us up to fail right from the start. They promise quick and immediate results—all you have to do is take a sketchy pill or follow an unrealistic diet.

Of course in the end, it won't work out and you'll be sad that you didn't get the results you expected to. Then a couple of weeks later, you'll see an advertisement for the next latest and greatest weight loss supplement, only this time it's guaranteed to work! You can probably guess where this going...

We need to stop looking for the quick fixes and gimmicks that we *know* don't work. Instead, we need to get back to a simpler and healthier way of eating. We need to eat in a way that leaves us feeling more energized instead of tired. And finally, we need to eat in a way that allows us to effortlessly burn fat so we can get and stay lean. Essentially, we need to combine the health and fat burning benefits of the vegan and ketogenic diets together.

When teamed up, these two diets have the power to give you an amazingly healthy lifestyle, and you'll be looking better than you ever have before. Here are a few of the main things you'll learn from this book:

- What the vegan and ketogenic diets are
- The health and weight loss benefits they'll provide to you
- A solid exercise routine you can follow
- How to set up and get your vegan and ketogenic diet started
- 53 vegan and ketogenic friendly recipes

Let's jump right in and get started!

Chapter 1: It's Time to Take Back Control of Our Health

Have you ever eaten a meal before that consisted mostly of sugar and junk food? How did you feel afterwards? I know for myself, whenever I eat a bunch of sugary foods at parties I feel pretty bad afterwards! Compare that feeling to how you feel after completing a workout or eating a healthy meal. You feel energized, amped up, and ready to go, right?

Imagine if you lived your life in a complete fog, drinking coffee throughout the day in order to stay awake and function. You could barely walk up a flight of stairs without being out of breath. Sadly, this is how many Americans are living their lives today! Most people never realize that they're in a daze, or that they could take actionable steps that would make them feel so much better and alive.

The first and most important step of any nutrition plan is to realize that you *can* change. Regardless of the decisions you've made in the past, or how unhealthy you've been in the past, you can still change. You must take responsibly for your health and well being, starting right now. Nothing is going to fall from the sky and make you change. No one is going to force you to change. It must come from within you.

If your mental image of yourself is that you're overweight and unhealthy, then what are your chances of succeeding? Probably not that high! You must begin to change the way you view yourself by changing your actions. And I get it, changing your habits and actions aren't easy. If it were easy, then everyone would be in great shape. Instead, it's far easier to sit on the couch, binge watch T.V., and eat junk food.

Once you've made up your mind and decided that you will become healthy and fit, no matter what, you must prepare yourself for other people who will unintentionally or intentionally try to sabotage your results.

Think about all of the food companies out there that produce junk food. All they care about is getting you addicted to their salty and sugary junk food so they can profit off you for a long time to come! Do you think they care about your long-term health and longevity? Not a chance!

Your friends and family may get in your way as well. They probably won't understand your reasoning behind going on a vegan keto diet, and how it can help to improve your health. It can also be easy to give into social pressure and norms at parties when everyone else is eating as freely as they please.

You must always remember the bigger picture and why you started down this path in the first place. Ultimately, you're the one who's in control of your own health. Don't let anyone else get in the way of that. As long as you remember that, you will stay on path and achieve your health goals.

The overall point of this book isn't to simply tell you about the vegan keto diet, but to make you successful with the diet. I want to help you get the lasting results you deserve instead of you fizzling out with the diet after a couple of weeks.

Chapter 2: What is the Ketogenic Diet?

The ketogenic diet is a low-carb, high-fat, and moderate protein diet. The main premise behind the diet is to make your body more efficient at using fat for fuel instead of sugar. When you're consuming a lot of carbohydrates, your body's blood sugar levels will spike up. Your body will then release a hormone called insulin to help regulate your blood sugar back down to normal. Here are the two main functions of insulin:

1. To tell fat cells to produce and store fat, and to hold on to the fat they already carry.
2. To pick up glucose from the bloodstream and burn that glucose instead of fat.

What it boils down to is that insulin fuels lipolysis, which is the burning of fat; insulin also fuels lipogenesis, which is the production of fat. Needless to say, insulin is very important to be in control of if you want to burn fat! Remember, the second function of insulin is to burn off glucose in the bloodstream instead of fat. This means that if you're eating a lot of carbs, your body will be focusing on burning off those carbs rather than fat. Unfortunately, your body doesn't burn *any* fat when insulin levels are spiked (8).

This makes sense because carbs are your body's first source of energy (9), so it'll tap into that first and then go to your fat stores. Of course, that's not what we want! In a perfect world, we would get to choose for our bodies to use fat for fuel as its first source of energy, but sadly it doesn't work that way. Instead, we must keep our insulin levels low by lowering our carbohydrate intake, and then our bodies will be forced to burn fat for fuel instead of carbs.

Luckily, this is where the ketogenic diet really shines. By following a ketogenic diet, you'll lower your carbs enough to put your body in a metabolic state known as ketosis. When you're in a state of ketosis, your body becomes way more efficient at burning fat for fuel instead of carbohydrates (10). The name of the game with the ketogenic diet is to stay in a state of ketosis for as long as you can!

Different Ways to Do the Ketogenic Diet

Believe it or not, there are actually quite a few different ways out there you can do the ketogenic diet based on your individual needs:

Standard Ketogenic Diet: this is the most common and most popular version of the ketogenic diet, and it's the one we'll mostly be focusing on. It involves consuming around 75% of your calories from fat, 20% from protein, and the remaining 5% from carbs.

Targeted Ketogenic Diet: with this type of ketogenic diet, you'll add in carbs before and after your workouts. Other than that, everything else is the same as the standard keto diet. Typically you'll consume around .33 grams of carbs per pound of bodyweight before and after your workout. For most people, this will equate to roughly 40-80 grams of carbs per meal. Pre and post workout carbohydrates have been shown to increase performance and aid in recovery (11). Therefore, if you're an athlete or an individual who trains with a lot of intensity on a regular basis, this type of ketogenic diet is for you.

Cyclical Ketogenic Diet: this is more of an advanced type of ketogenic diet. With this style of keto, you'll devote one or two full days to eating high carbohydrates in order to refill muscle glycogen stores. You'll usually consume around 50%

of your total calories from carbs on these days. This will help to promote muscle growth for athletes or individuals looking to build muscle. A proper workout routine (which will be covered later) must be in place in order for you to fully deplete your muscle glycogen stores. If not, you could end up gaining a little bit of body fat. Due to the precise planning and fact that's it's easy to overeat on your high-carb days, this version of keto isn't recommended for beginners.

High-Protein Ketogenic Diet: this style of ketogenic diet is similar to the standard ketogenic diet, except that it contains more protein and less fat. Typically you'll eat around 60% fat, 35% protein, and 5% carbs with this type of ketogenic diet. This style is great for individuals who engage regularly in vigorous activity and want a higher protein intake to help prevent muscle loss. Protein is also very satiating and will help to keep you fuller for a longer period of time when your calories are being restricted.

For the purposes of this book, we'll be focusing our attention mostly on the standard ketogenic diet. This version of the ketogenic diet is backed by the most research and it's the easiest for beginners to get started with.

Foods to Avoid:

Eating low carbs might seem easy enough to do on the surface, but many people struggle with knowing exactly what constitutes a low-carb food vs. a high-carb food. Carbs are contained in many different foods that you may not realize. The best thing you can do if you're unsure is to look it up online and see how many carbs a certain food actually contains.

Later on, I'll be providing you with some keto friendly recipes that you can use while on the diet. For now however, I want to provide you with a list of foods that you'll need to avoid eating while on the ketogenic diet. These are foods that are high in sugar or carbs and will take you out of ketosis. Here's the list:

Grains: any wheat-based product such as rice, cereal, pasta, etc.

Fruit: yes fruit is healthy for you, however for the purposes of the ketogenic diet it's not allowed because fruit contains fructose and that will take your body out of ketosis.

Sugary foods: this would include things such as fruit juice, smoothies, ice cream, cookies, candy, soda, diet soda, and other sugar-free diet foods. Sugar-free foods usually contain sugar alcohols, which can affect ketone levels.

Alcohol: alcoholic drinks contain a high amount of carbs and can kick you out of ketosis.

Unhealthy fats: yes, the ketogenic diet is a high fat diet, however you want to be consuming healthy fats. Avoid processed vegetable oils and trans fat.

Low-Fat products: many low-fat food items are either high in sugar or carbs to replace the fat content and should be avoided.

Beans: yes most beans are healthy, but the high-carb content will ruin the benefits of the diet. Avoid eating any type of bean including: peas, lentils, chickpeas, black beans, kidney beans, etc.

Root Vegetables: you might be thinking, "What? I thought vegetables were good for you!" Yes, vegetables certainly are good for you, but particular vegetables are higher in carbs and will do more harm than good while on a ketogenic diet. Don't consume potatoes, sweet potatoes, carrots, turnips, etc.

Foods to Eat

The list of foods to avoid is quite large, and it might leave you wondering what you can eat on a ketogenic diet. Luckily, there are still plenty of foods you can eat that will provide plenty of variety so you'll never get bored constantly eating the same foods over and over:

Eggs: eggs are a great source of protein and fat, and they contain no carbs. It's a versatile food that can be made in a lot of different dishes.

Cheese: cheese gets a bad rep for being unhealthy, but it's a very keto-friendly food. It contains virtually no carbs and will help you reach your daily fat intake.

Nuts: various nuts such as almonds, cashews, peanuts, etc. contain healthy fats and are a great snack choice if you're on the go a lot.

Seeds: pumpkin seeds, chia seeds, flax seeds, etc. are high in fiber and can easily be thrown into many dishes without changing the taste of the recipe.

Healthy Oils: similar to seeds, healthy oils such as olive oil and coconut oil can be added seamlessly to dishes without a noticeable difference in taste.

Low-Carb Vegetables: not all vegetables are excluded from the ketogenic diet. Any leafy green vegetable can be eaten along with onions and peppers without worry of exceeding your carb limit.

Butter: Similar to cheese, butter tends to get labeled as unhealthy. However, when it comes to butter, the quality and kind you get matters big time. Stay away from the margarine and buy grass-fed if you can.

Avocados: makes for great guacamole and avocados are a healthy fat. Enough said.

Chapter 3: Health Benefits of the Ketogenic Diet

Research has shown the ketogenic diet to be a great way to lose weight (12). That's cool and all, but losing weight shouldn't be the only thing you seek with a diet. You should have more energy, and better indications of health such as lower cholesterol. Starting a ketogenic diet can provide you with some amazing health benefits in addition to losing weight:

Prevention of diabetes: diabetes is essentially an impaired function of insulin. Studies have shown the ketogenic diet to be able to improve insulin sensitivity (13). The higher your insulin sensitivity levels are, the less insulin your body will require to lower blood glucose levels back to normal. As you learned in the previous chapter, your body doesn't burn fat when insulin levels are high. Therefore, it's important to improve insulin sensitivity levels to help better regulate blood glucose levels.

Lower Risk for Heart disease: heart disease is one of the leading causes of death in the United States, and it includes many risk factors such as cholesterol levels, body fat, blood sugar, and blood pressure. The ketogenic diet can help to improve these risk factors, thus lowering the risk for heart disease (14).

Getting rid of acne: another cool side benefit is that it can help get rid of acne if you struggle with breakouts regularly. The ketogenic diet will help to lower insulin levels by eating less processed foods and sugar, which can help prevent acne.

Cancer treatment: the ketogenic diet is currently being used to treat several different types of cancer, and it can slow tumor growth (15). Of course, more research needs to be done for conclusive evidence.

Increase HDL cholesterol levels: there are two different kinds of cholesterol—HDL, which stands for high-density lipoproteins and LDL, which stands for low-density lipoproteins. Your HDL is your good cholesterol that you want to increase because it's responsible for carrying cholesterol to the liver where it can then be excreted or reused. LDL's on the other hand, are bad cholesterol, and are responsible for carrying cholesterol away from the liver and into the body. Research shows one of the best ways to increase your HDL levels are to increase your fat intake (16). You'll easily be able to achieve that with the standard ketogenic protocol of 75% of your calories coming from fat.

Lower blood pressure: Lowering your carbohydrate intake has been shown to decrease hypertension (17). Having higher blood pressure increases your risk for developing diseases such as heart disease and stroke.

Decrease triglyceride levels: triglycerides are a fat molecule. It might sound counter-intuitive that increasing your fat intake would decrease the amount of triglycerides in the blood, but it really does. This occurs because carbs are one of the biggest contributors to increasing triglycerides (18). Therefore, by decreasing carb intake, you'll decrease the amount of triglycerides in your blood.

More weight loss than a typical diet: Studies have shown that people who restrict calories on a low-carb diet lose more weight, and lose weight faster than individuals restricting calories on a low-fat diet (19). The main reason for this is because low-carb diets lower insulin levels, which will cause the body to get rid of excess sodium within the first few weeks of starting the diet.

A positive way to lose your appetite: When you go on a diet and restrict your calories, you start to feel hungry. If your feelings of hunger start to get out of control, you're more likely to quit and give up on your diet—and obviously if you quit and go back to your old habits, you have no chance of losing weight and improving your health. Luckily, eating a low-carb diet has been shown to decrease appetite (20). This is critical because it'll allow you to lower your overall caloric intake without having to worry about getting extra hungry.

Chapter 4: What is a Vegan Lifestyle?

When I was a kid, I would regularly get in trouble for trying to talk to my mom while she was on the phone. I had no idea who she was talking to or what it was about, all I knew was that what I had to say was the number one priority. If I wanted more juice, she needed to drop everything and tend to my needs!

Being older, I now understand that whatever my mom was doing on the phone was way more important than what I needed. I also understand that it's rude to interrupt someone while they're on the phone. However, when I was a little kid, I had no idea of that concept whatsoever. I couldn't comprehend another person's perspective, only my own. Getting more juice was the only thing that mattered to me in that moment!

The same can be said for many people and their understanding of veganism. It doesn't make sense to a lot of people that someone would become vegan. They don't understand the health benefits that it can provide. They don't think it's possible to get enough protein or certain vitamins.

Similar to when I was a kid, they simply don't comprehend the other person's perspective, and they're likely uneducated about veganism. Therefore, when starting a vegan diet, it's important to know up front that other people might question why you're on this certain type of diet. Don't get frustrated by their lack of knowledge, instead use the time to educate them on the benefits that a vegan diet can provide.

What is Veganism and How Did It All Get Started?

There are quite a few different types of vegans. A dietary vegan is someone who abstains from animal products strictly with diet. This would mean that you wouldn't eat anything that was made using animals. However, veganism can also extend beyond simply diet and include ethical and environmental vegans as well.

Ethical vegans are against the use of animals for any reason whatsoever. They don't buy or use any products that are made using animals. This would include things such as fur rugs or coats, leather, soap made from tallow, etc.

Environmental vegans are similar to ethical vegans, except they don't use animal products because they believe that industrial farming is bad for the environment and is unsustainable. For the purposes of this book, we'll focus on dietary veganism.

In terms of the history of veganism, it's not that old of an idea—less than 100 years believe it or not. The word vegan first came about from a man named Donald Watson. He cofounded the Vegan Society in England, and this group still exists today.

The people who founded this society wanted to do more than only avoid eating meat. They decided to eliminate not just meat, but dairy and eggs as well—and veganism was born. Not only did the Vegan society not eat any foods made from animals, but they clarified early on that they didn't use any animal products. So from the beginning, people of the Vegan Society didn't view veganism as something relating strictly to diet.

Since the 1940's veganism has increased in popularity, particularly since 2010. It's easy to see why. We live in the information era. In today's world, it's so much easier to spread knowledge around than it was when veganism first started in 1944. Today, we have access to eBooks, articles, and online videos that we can access instantly to learn about any given topic.

So needless to say, if people want to learn about veganism, they can easily do so. However, 70 plus years ago most people had never even heard about veganism or knew what it was. Today, although most people may have heard about veganism, they might not know much about it, or be willing to learn more about it.

In addition to information and knowledge being spread more, we also see more restaurants offering vegan options, and a bigger expansion of vegan-friendly foods in grocery stores. In 2012, it was estimated that approximately 2% of the U.S. population was vegan (16). That might not seem like a lot, but that still equates to roughly 6.3 million vegans in the U.S. alone.

Common Misconceptions About a Vegan Diet

There are plenty of myths that surround a vegan diet, but here are a few of the most common ones:

Myth #1: You can't get enough protein on a vegan diet

This is definitely the most common thing vegans will hear about their diet. People associate protein with meat and think that the only way someone could get enough protein in their diet is by eating meat. There are plenty of options you have to get in enough protein as a vegan:

- Quinoa
- Chickpeas
- Beans
- Tempeh
- Tofu
- Hemp

Myth #2: Vegan Diets Are Too Expensive

Many people think that eating healthy food such as leafy green vegetables is too expensive. Usually though, these people just want to make up excuses for continuing to eat their unhealthy diet. Foods like beans, fruits, vegetables, rice, and other vegan staples are not as expensive as buying meat is. And some of these food items like rice and beans have a much longer shelf life than meat does.

Myth #3: You Need to Eat Meat to Be Healthy

There is research to show that eating a vegan diet can reduce your risk for heart disease and type 2 diabetes (17). A vegan diet can also lower your cholesterol and blood pressure as well (18). Case in point—you don't need meat to be healthy.

Myth #4: You Can't Get Enough Calcium on a Vegan Diet

This is another argument similar to the one about not being able to get enough protein. However, milk and cheese aren't the only sources of calcium. You can get plenty of calcium from foods like kale, spinach, and figs, among others.

Myth #5: You'll Be Hungry a Lot

This idea comes from people who eat meat and think that's the only way you can have a filling and satisfying meal. How could you possibly get full eating vegetables? Well, it's actually quite easy! Many foods you'll be eating on a vegan diet are rich in fiber, which will help to keep you fuller longer. Beans and leafy green vegetables are rich in fiber, making it hard not to get and stay full!

Chapter 5: Health Benefits of a Vegan Diet

There are many health benefits that a vegan diet will provide to you. The typical American diet today isn't a very good one. Many people eat fast food on a daily basis, and they eat way too many unhealthy fats and simple sugars.

It's way more convenient to drive through and get fast food after a long day of work instead of preparing a healthy meal. It's unfortunate that approximately 610,000 Americans die from heart disease each year (19), and most of these deaths could have been prevented with a proper diet and exercise routine. Yes going on a vegan diet isn't going to be the easiest thing in the world to do, but the gained health benefits are worth it.

There are many restaurants you won't be able to eat at. You'll have to plan ahead for parties and other events that likely won't have vegan-friendly options. With all of that being said though, you must remember why you started a vegan diet in the first place. Being vegan won't be easy at times, and if you lose sight of the reason why you started the diet in the first place, then you'll be more likely to give up on the diet.

Here are some of the common reasons why people start a vegan diet in the first place:

Helps with the Environment

When many people think about going green or saving the planet, they typically think about recycling more or reducing the use of plastic. That's a great start, but becoming a vegan can do more than you might think. One of the main reasons for this is because the livestock segment is the biggest producer of nitrous oxide and methane gases. Many people think that carbon dioxide is the worst gas that contributes the most to climate change, but it's actually methane and nitrous oxide.

While carbon dioxide may not be the most damaging gas for climate change, it still has an impact, and approximately 9% of carbon dioxide emission in the United States comes from the livestock segment (20).

Another factor that many people don't take into consideration when it comes to livestock and the environment is deforestation. Think about it—if you're going to herd all of the animals together and keep them in one place, you need large areas of land for them to live on. This can make a lot of forests disappear, which can trigger climate change and destroy a lot of natural habitats for animals living in the forests.

Kind Regards for Animals

When I was in high school, one of my friends was in a youth organization that raised animals and then showed them off in competition. Depending on how well your animal would place, you would get to sell it for a certain amount of money. He had gotten a pig and started raising it from a young age for the competition.

After a while of feeding and playing with the pig everyday, he eventually became emotionally attached to the animal. It was very difficult for him to let go of the pig after the competition, but that's what he had to do. The pig of course was sent off, slaughtered, and later eaten. He didn't eat any meat products made from pigs for a year after that happened, just to ensure he wouldn't eat his own pig.

You don't have to raise your own pig to feel sympathy for these animals. There are many non-vegan and non-vegetarians out there who would still feel bad or sick if they watched the slaughtering of an animal. By going on a vegan diet, you can help save animals everywhere. To put things into perspective, this is the amount of pounds of meat produced for the month of August in 2017 (21):

- Commercial Red Meat Production: 4.63 billion pounds
- Beef Production: 2.4 billion pounds
- Veal Production: 6.4 million pounds
- Pork Production: 2.21 billion pounds
- Lamb and Mutton Production: 12.8 million pounds

As you can see, these numbers are quite high, and you might be thinking to yourself, "How can one person going vegan make a difference?" Well that's similar to the attitude of, "Why should I vote? My one vote won't change the outcome of the election?" Imagine if everyone thought like that though. What if no one voted because they believed that their single vote didn't matter? Then all of the sudden any single person's vote would matter greatly!

Ultimately, it's not about the single vote or a single person going vegan. It's about the principle behind it. It's about standing up for what you believe in and focusing on what you're in control of. Sure, you can't make everyone become a vegan, but you can be a good living example of a vegan for the people that are around you.

They'll see how much you care, and they'll be able to tell how passionate you are about animals. They might get curious and ask questions, or possibly even become vegan themselves one day. You'll never know unless you try!

To Help Improve Your Health
And finally one of the main reasons why people become vegan is for the amazing health benefits that the diet can

provide to you. People who regularly follow a vegan diet have a lower risk for the following diseases:

- Decreased risk for heart disease by 26-68%
- Decreased risk for prostate cancer by 35%
- Decreased risk for type 2 diabetes by 25-49%
- Decreased risk for hypertension by 55%

These numbers should come as a big relief considering how unhealthy many Americans are today. Approximately 1 in every 4 males and 1 in every 5 females in the U.S. die from cancer (22), and about 1 out of every 3 Americans has high blood pressure (23).

Here are some other benefits you'll likely experience by starting a vegan diet:

1. Better for Weight Loss

Studies have shown that going on a plant-based type of diet can help you lose more weight than individuals not on a plant-based diet (24). This is because going on a plant-based diet such as veganism means you'll be consuming more natural, unprocessed foods. These foods are not only healthier for you, but also they typically contain fewer calories than the processed junk food that many people are eating today.

The reason for this is that wholesome foods like fruits and vegetables are nutrient dense and they have a low caloric density. Nutrient density refers to the amount of vitamins and minerals that are in a food relative to its weight. Caloric density refers to the amount of calories that are in a food based on its weight. Processed foods have a low nutrient density and a high caloric density. So, not only do they have a high amount of calories, but also they won't do a very good job of filling you up because of their low nutrient profile.

Imagine eating 100 calories worth of vegetables versus eating 100 calories worth of candy. You would have to eat way more of the vegetables to reach that 100-calorie mark than you would the candy. Not only that, but the vegetables will provide your body with so many healthy vitamins and minerals, while the candy will only give you a sugar rush. Finally, you won't be hungry soon after eating the vegetables, but the candy will do little to fill you up.

This is something very important to think about because it's not solely the excess calories in junk food that kills you—it's also the lack of fiber and nutrients, among other things. This'll cause you to go back and eat more soon after your meal, simply because it didn't meet your body's nutritional demands.

2. Improve Digestive Health

There are quite a few fruits and vegetables that contain a good amount of prebiotics and probiotics. Prebiotics are non-digestible carbs that perform as fuel for probiotics. Prebiotics act in a symbiotic relationship when combined with probiotics.

Think of prebiotics as the sidekick to any superhero. Sure, the superhero is powerful on his own, but the sidekick comes in handy, and is even necessary to stop evil at times. Probiotics on the other hand, are a type of beneficial bacteria that live in different organs, and their main function is to help aid in digestion.

Of course it's great to consume more of the healthy nutrients that our bodies need. However, it's not how many nutrients you eat that matters—it's how many nutrients your body digests and absorbs that ultimately makes the difference. Therefore, you can consume all of the healthy foods you want, but your body must be able to properly digest, absorb, and use the vitamins and minerals from that food. If it can't, then the food you ate might not be as healthy as it appeared.

This is why it's critical to consume more foods that contain large amounts of prebiotics and probiotics. Here's a list of a few things you can eat on a vegan diet that contain a healthy amount of either prebiotics or probiotics:

- Cultured vegetables, like kimchi or sauerkraut. (One of my personal favorites. Can you blame me? I have German heritage.)
- Kombucha
- Apple cider vinegar
- Coconut kefir
- Olives
- Miso
- Tempeh

Consuming more of these types of foods will help to line your digestive track with more healthy bacteria, which will aid in absorption of key nutrients from the other foods you consume.

3. Increase in Other Helpful Substances Such As Enzymes and Antioxidants

When you want to get and stay healthy, eating wholesome foods is a great start, but it's not everything. You need a complete defense to help protect you from disease as much as possible.

This is where enzymes and antioxidants can come into play. Being on a vegan diet will allow you to consume more fresh fruits and vegetables, and if you're consuming a lot of this produce raw, you can consume even more antioxidants and enzymes.

Enzymes are a substance that acts as a catalyst to bring about a certain biochemical reaction. That science-y definition probably sounds like a mouthful, so let me break it down for you; enzymes enable your body to break down food particles into usable nutrients. Therefore, the more usable enzymes a food contains, the easier it'll be to digest and process. This is why it's important to eat your produce raw when appropriate because the cooking process destroys many of the enzymes found in the food.

Antioxidants seem equally as complicated as enzymes. They remove potentially damaging oxidizing agents in a living organism. In other words—we need antioxidants to help prevent cell damage caused by oxidants. And because our bodies are made up of tons of individual cells, it's important to keep them healthy and protected.

Here's a list of some foods that contain a good amount of antioxidants:

- Kiwis
- Pumpkin
- Blueberries
- Cranberries
- Kidney beans
- Pecans
- Goji berries

Eating more foods like these by starting a vegan diet will help to prevent disease and help combat against free radicals in the body like oxidants.

4. Prevention of Syndrome X

Syndrome X is commonly referred to as metabolic syndrome, and approximately 47 million Americans have it (25). That's a staggering 1 out of every 6 Americans! Syndrome X itself isn't a disease; it's a collection of risk factors that increase the likelihood for heart disease, stroke, and diabetes.

Here are the factors:

- Blood sugar: 100 mg/dL or higher

- Blood pressure: 135/85 mm Hg or higher
- Large Waist: Over 40 inches for men and 35 inches for women
- High Amounts of Bad Cholesterol: 150 mg/dL or higher
- Low Amounts of Good Cholesterol: Less than 40 mg/dL for men and less than 50 mg/dL for women

You have to have at least 3 of these risk factors to be diagnosed with syndrome X. By consuming more wholesome foods with a vegan diet, you can help to greatly reduce your risk for developing any of these harmful diseases associated with metabolic syndrome.

5. Helps with Osteoporosis and Arthritis

Osteoporosis is a disease in which the density and quality of the bones in the body is reduced. Anyone can develop osteoporosis, however women are more than 4 times as likely to develop osteoporosis than men (26). This is because the ovaries stop producing a key hormone called oestrogen once a woman goes through menopause.

At first glance though, it wouldn't appear that a vegan diet would be good for osteoporosis. When you think of strong bones, you usually think about calcium. In a typical American diet, people get most of their calcium from sources like cheese and milk. You can't eat those foods on a vegan diet, which is why most people would think that a vegan diet is bad for osteoporosis.

Upon further inspection however, there are plenty of vegan-friendly foods that are high in calcium:

- Kale
- Spinach
- Figs
- Turnip Greens
- Black-Eyed Peas

- Almond Milk

Another misconception about bone health is that only calcium matters. There are plenty of other vitamins that help make bones strong such as vitamins D and K, magnesium, and potassium. Eating various types of beans, leafy greens, and even getting some exposure to the sun will help you get plenty of these key vitamins.

Arthritis is an inflammation that occurs within one or more joints and causes pain and stiffness that can worsen with age. Research is being done showing how a probiotic-rich vegan diet can help with the symptoms of arthritis such as pain, morning stiffness, and joint swelling when compared to people eating an omnivorous diet (27).

Chapter 6: Why Combine a Vegan and Ketogenic Diet?

When I first started working out, I wanted to achieve all of my fitness goals at once:

- Get a six-pack
- Dunk a basketball
- Build muscle
- Run faster
- Increase endurance

And by chasing all of these rabbit holes, I ended up achieving none of my goals. Looking back on it, I realized that it's better to focus on achieving one goal at a time before moving onto the next. In my case, I would need to dunk a basketball before moving onto trying to lean down to get a six-pack. Then once I got ripped six-pack abs, I would try to accomplish another goal, such as increasing endurance.

Why then should you try to combine a vegan diet with the ketogenic diet? Won't you be spreading yourself too thin and end up not achieving anything like I did when I first started working out? The answer is no because veganism and the ketogenic diet work synergistically together to achieve one common goal—fat loss and better health. My problem was that I wanted to achieve varying goals that contrasted one another.

For example, I wanted to build muscle and burn fat at the same time. Yes, this is possible for beginners to pull off, but it usually complicates things. This is because in order for you to build muscle, you need to be in a caloric surplus by consuming more calories than you burn off. And in order for you to burn fat, you need to be in a caloric deficit by burning off more calories than you consume (I'll go more in depth on surpluses and deficits later). Since you can't be in a surplus and a deficit at the same time, can you see how these contradictory goals can complicate things?

I tried heading in one direction to build muscle, and then I would turn around and go in the opposite direction to try and burn fat. In the end, I stayed exactly where I was at and went nowhere. Keep things simple and go for one goal at a time. Lose all of the weight that you want, and then start trying to build muscle.

Fortunately, it's easy to combine a vegan diet with the ketogenic diet to maximize the health and weight loss benefits. All you'll need to do is start with either the ketogenic diet or the vegan diet. Once you're comfortable with the original diet you chose (which will usually take about 2 weeks), you'll simply add in the other diet and combine it with the original diet. For example, let's say you decided to start the ketogenic diet first. You would solely follow the ketogenic diet for 2 weeks, and then you would add in the vegan diet with the ketogenic diet.

This is the optimal way to do things because immediately jumping into a vegan ketogenic diet can be too much too soon, which will cause you to crash and burn. By starting one diet, getting used to it, and then adding in the other diet, you'll set yourself up for a much smoother transition.

The main reason why these diets work so well together is because you can use the ketogenic diet to help you burn fat, and you can use the vegan diet to help you stay healthy. Sure, the ketogenic diet has its health benefits, and it's possible to lose weight with a vegan diet, but those aren't their strengths. The ketogenic diet is great for burning fat because of the low-carb and high fat intake.

This will help to put your body in a state that I mentioned earlier called ketosis. And ketosis is definitely something you'll want to take advantage of because it'll make your body use fat for fuel instead of carbohydrates. Of course on its own, a vegan diet won't put your body in a state of ketosis. However, a vegan diet will provide you with specific health benefits that a ketogenic diet won't. Combining both of these diets will allow each diet to play off of the other's weakness.

A common question people have is, "How many meals should I eat per day?" There's a popular myth that states that eating more frequently helps to boost your metabolism, which would mean that eating smaller, more frequent meals will allow you to lose more weight. Research shows that this actually isn't the case. Studies have shown that meal frequency does nothing to boost metabolism and aid with weight loss (28).

Feel free to eat as often as you like. If you want to eat a standard breakfast, lunch, and dinner, then go for it. Eating 1-2 or as many as 6 meals a day is perfectly okay as well. Eat in a way that fits best with your schedule and lifestyle. You need to be more focused with *what* you're eating, not how often you're eating.

Chapter 7: Setting Up Your Vegan Ketogenic Diet

Here's the exact step-by-step process you need to take to set up your vegan keto diet:

Step #1: Understand the Importance of Calories

You've undoubtedly heard of the word calorie before. But what exactly is a calorie? Is it something evil you should avoid whenever possible? Is it the bane of your existence?

Some people have an idea of what a calorie is, but most don't know. If you went out on the street and asked 10 different people what a calorie is, you'd likely get 10 different answers. Here's the textbook definition of a calorie:

"The energy needed to raise the temperature of 1 gram of water through 1° C"

Sounds complicated right? Essentially, a calorie is a measurement of energy. Your body is constantly undergoing chemical reactions to keep you alive. All of these chemical reactions (digestion, breathing, organ function, etc.) require energy.

Your body gets the energy necessary to continue functioning from the food (calories) you eat. Calories aren't your worst enemy; they're your friend. You have to work with them, not against them. And as you're about to find out, not all calories are the same.

Is a Calorie a Calorie?

This is a big debate in the fitness industry. If I eat 100 calories from a candy bar, and you eat 100 calories worth of vegetables, are we equal? Well, yes and no.

One calorie *is* one calorie regardless of what source the calorie came from. Trying to argue with this is like saying one yard going east isn't the same distance as going one yard west. The difference lies in the *macronutrient* quality.

100 calories from vegetables and 100 calories from candy is still 100 calories. Both are made up mostly of carbs; the quality of those carbs is what makes them very different. The candy contains simple carbs and sugar.

It won't provide you with any vitamins, nutrients, or fiber. It also won't be very satiating. The vegetables, on the other hand, are complex carbs.

They'll provide you with quality complex carbs and a good source of vitamins, nutrients, and fiber. Additionally, nutritious food like fruits and vegetables will keep you fuller longer, which is critical during calorie restriction for weight loss purposes. Therefore, quality of calories can be just as important as quantity of calories.

The Caloric Deficit is King

Pop quiz: What's the *only* way your body can burn fat?

If you looked at the title above and guessed caloric deficit, then you'd be correct! A caloric deficit is simply when you burn off more calories than you consume. The opposite is a caloric surplus—consuming more calories than you burn off. And maintenance is when you are at a caloric equilibrium.

Here's an example:

-Joe burns 2,000 calories a day and eats 1,800. He's in a caloric deficit of 200 calories, and he'll start to lose weight.
-Joe burns 2,000 calories a day and eats 2,200. He's in a caloric surplus of 200 calories, and he'll start to gain weight.
-Joe burns 2,000 calories a day and eats 2,000. He's at maintenance and will not gain or lose weight.

Starting a vegan keto diet isn't enough to guarantee results. It's still possible for you to overeat on healthy fats and not lose any weight. It's also possible for you to eat too little and crash and burn because you're hungry all of the time. That's why you must know the numbers behind exactly how much you need to eat in order to lose weight. The vegan keto diet will structure *how* you eat, but determining your resting metabolic rate in the next step will determine the *amount* you need to eat to start burning fat.

Step #2: Determine Your Resting Metabolic Rate

As I mentioned earlier, every day your body needs energy (calories) in order to continue on with all of its chemical functions such as breathing, digesting food, organ function, etc. The amount of calories you burn in any given day is your resting metabolic rate (rmr). Once you figure out your body's rmr, you can then determine how many calories you need to eat to start burning fat.

Determining your rmr is simple—multiply your bodyweight in pounds by 13.
Let's use myself as an example:

Body Weight=200 pounds
200 x 13= RMR of 2,600

This means that if I eat less than 2,600 calories I'll be in a caloric deficit and I'll start to lose weight. If I eat more than 2,600 calories I'll be in a caloric surplus and I'll start to gain weight. And finally, if I eat exactly 2,600 calories, I'll be at maintenance and I'll neither gain nor lose weight.

The question is—how big of a caloric deficit do you need to create in order for it to translate into pounds lost? There's about 3,500 calories in one pound of fat (29), meaning that you must create a cumulative caloric deficit of 3,500 calories in order to lose 1 pound. So if you divide 3,500 by 7 days in a week, you'll need to create an average daily caloric deficit of 500 calories to lose 1 pound per week.

Referring back to the example from above, here's what that would translate to:

RMR- 2,600 − 500= 2,100

This means that I need to eat 2,100 calories everyday if I want to lose 1 pound per week. The more weight you have to lose, the larger the caloric deficit you can create. For example, you could eat at a caloric deficit of 750 calories and lose 1.5 pounds per week, or you could eat at a deficit of 1,000 calories to lose 2 pounds per week.

Essentially, for every 250 calories you can expect to lose an additional .5-pound. The key is to not get carried away. You might want to lose all of the weight as soon as possible and jump right into a 1,000-calorie caloric deficit.

That may not be the best idea. For most people, losing 1 pound per week by creating a 500-calorie caloric deficit is golden. Imagine yourself a year from now being 52 pounds lighter without having to put forth much effort! That's much better than spinning your wheels trying to lose 100 pounds in that same time frame.

Step #3: Set Up Your Macro Percentages

In case you're unfamiliar, a macro is simply a protein, carb, or fat. And now we're going to figure out exactly how many grams of carbs, protein, and fat you need to be eating on a daily basis. From there, you'll simply eat that much and start seeing results. It really is that simple.

Before we can get into the specifics of each macro, it's critical that you know what your resting metabolic rate is by multiplying your bodyweight by 13.

Then if you want to lose weight, subtract 500 from your RMR. This is the total amount of calories you'll eat on a daily basis.

Once you know that information, you can move onto the next section.

Setting Up Your Macro Percentages

The first thing we must determine is the percentage of our diet each macronutrient (protein, carb, and fat) will make up. Since we're following a standard ketogenic diet, these are the percentages we'll use:

- Protein: 20% of total calories
- Carbs: 5% of total calories
- Fat: 75% of total calories

Note: You can also try the cyclical ketogenic diet instead of the standard ketogenic diet if you want to have more flexibility with your carbs. This'll make things easier to enjoy certain vegan staples such as beans, rice, and various fruits. With the cyclical ketogenic diet, you'll consume 50% of your total calories from carbs twice per week. I recommend following the same macro percentages from the standard keto diet on your low-carb days (5% carbs, 20% protein, and 75% fat). Of course, you don't have to eat 50% of your calories from carbs if you don't want to. The idea is to provide you with more flexibility with your carb intake, so feel free to only consume 30-40% carbs if needed on those days.

Here's what your percentages look like if you choose to do a cyclical ketogenic diet:

- Protein: 20% of total calories
- Carbs: 50% of total calories
- Fat: 30% of total calories

Side Note: If you want to eat less carbs, add the leftover percent to your fat intake. For example, if you're going to eat only 30% carbs on your high-carb days, then eat 50% fat and keep protein at 20%.

Now that you know the total amount of calories you need to eat, and you know the percentage for each macro, we can determine how many calories of protein, carbs, and fat you'll need to eat. Before we do though, it's important to remember the following:

Number of calories per gram of protein=4
Number of calories per gram of carb=4
Number of calories per gram of fat=9

I'll use myself as an example again:

Resting metabolic rate=2,600 calories

If I want to burn fat:

2,600-500=2,100 daily calories

2,100 x .20= 420 total daily calories from protein
2,100 x .05= 105 total daily calories from carbs
2,100 x .75= 1,575 total daily calories from fat

You can determine the grams equivalent of these total calorie numbers by doing the following:

420/4=105 grams of protein per day
105/4=26.25 grams of carbs per day

1,575/9=175 grams of fat per day

And for cyclical ketogenic diet on high carb days:

2,600-500=2,100 daily calories

2,100 x .20= 420 total daily calories from protein
2,100 x .50= 1,050 total daily calories from carbs
2,100 x .30= 630 total daily calories from fat

Gram equivalent for cyclical ketogenic diet on high carb days:

420/4=105 grams of protein per day
1,050/4=262.5 grams of carbs per day
630/9=70 grams of fat per day

Yes, these numbers are very exact; however, don't try to be perfect. The reality is that you'll rarely eat 26.25 grams of carbs spot on, so don't fret over it. Instead, try to get within 5%-10% of the numbers and you'll be fine.

Step #4: Set Up Your Ketogenic Diet Protocol

Once you have your macros setup, the next thing you need to do is implement your keto diet, assuming this is the diet you want to start first. (Flip steps 4 and 5 if you would rather start with the vegan diet and add in the ketogenic diet later.) You'll want to choose between the standard and cyclical ketogenic diets. Both have their pros and cons, so test out both and see which one works best for you and your schedule.

The standard keto diet stays true to the core of its cause, which is keeping carbs low and fat high so your body can remain in a state of ketosis. The cyclical keto diet on the other hand, won't keep your body in ketosis on your high-carb days, but it'll be much easier to implement with a vegan diet. This is because many staples that are allowed in a ketogenic diet, like cheese, aren't allowed on a vegan diet. A standard keto diet won't allow you to eat any carbs that are considered staples for a vegan diet like fruit, rice, beans, etc. This limits your options. Of course, it's still possible to eat a standard keto diet with a vegan diet, but your food choices for carbs will primarily be limited to leafy green vegetables. If you want more of a variety every with what you can eat for carbs, then try out the cyclical keto diet.

Remember that it's critical that you only start with one diet at a time.
You'll make things far easier on yourself instead of burning out from trying to do too much at once. All you need to do during this two-week period is follow the ketogenic diet as it's laid out. Don't worry about getting every single detail down pat; do your best to follow the diet, and see what you like about it.

Then once the two-weeks is up, you can start using the overall diet that includes the calories, macros, ketogenic diet, and vegan diet.

Step #5: Add in the Vegan Diet

Once you've gotten used to the ketogenic diet, it's time for the fun part. You're going to add in the vegan diet with the ketogenic diet you've already started.

At this point, most of the hard work is already done. You already know how many calories you need to eat, and your exact macro percentages as well. From here, all you have to do is avoid eating any food products made from animals. The ketogenic diet provides the structure for how much of each macro you'll eat, and the vegan diet tell you what foods you should eat.

Step #6: Measure and Adjust

You might be thinking, this sounds great and all, but how do I actually track and measure my calories and macro percentages? This is certainly the most tedious part of any diet, but remember what get measured gets managed. You must track and account for the calories you're eating or else you'll have no clue what direction you're heading in.

The easiest way to track your macros is to go to the app store, type in macro tracker, and download one of the many apps that will track your macros. Most of the apps cost a couple of dollars, but that's a small price to pay. You can type in the food you're eating and it'll tell you how many calories are contained in the food, as well as how much protein, carbs, and fat it has. Most of the apps even have a barcode scanner where you can take a picture of what you're eating, and it'll automatically add the macros towards your daily numbers.

You'll have your phone on you wherever you go, so if you eat at a restaurant, for example, you can track the macros and calories right then and there. If you decide not to use an app, you'll have to track your macros using nutritional labels or by searching the nutritional information online. From there, you'll have to calculate the numbers yourself and record it on a note app or with pen and paper, which is certainly not ideal.

The more inconvenient something is to do, the less likely you are to stick with it. The vegan keto diet is a great nutritional plan, but only if you're able to keep up with it for the long haul. You want to keep things as simple and easy as possible—spend a couple of bucks and indulge in a macro tracking app to take the load off your shoulders. It'll pay for itself many times over.

The other thing you'll need to get is a food scale. You can get one of these on Amazon for around $11. This'll allow you to figure out the number of grams in the foods you're eating and calculate the macros from there.

Once you've been doing this diet for a while, you'll eventually start to get a feel for how you need to eat in order to lose weight. You'll know the general macro contents of the meals you regularly eat. You'll be able to do the eyeball test and guess roughly how many calories are in the foods you're eating.

This is a skill that'll come with time. Be patient, and don't rush it—that's when you'll start overestimating your calories. Tracking everything as accurately as possible is the key to success with any nutritional approach that you do. Be diligent about your measuring, especially in the beginning, even though it's quite tedious.

It might even take you a couple of weeks to get used to measuring and recording everything that you eat and drink. Be patient with yourself if it takes a few weeks for you to start seeing results. You'll get better and better with the process as time goes on. Nobody is a master at something the first time they do it.

One common question people have with this topic is, "How close do I have to be with my macro percentages and calories?" The reality is that you'll never be 100% spot on accurate with your numbers. Using the example from earlier, you'll never eat exactly 26.25 grams of carbs each day, and that's ok. You'll want to aim to be within 5-10% of what I recommend. For example, one day you might intake 65% of your diet from fat and 30% from protein. It's not worth the extra stress of getting every little number exactly right—you'll drive yourself nuts. You want to generally be as consistent and accurate as you possibly can.

The other thing you'll want to do is measure your weight. One mistake a lot of people make is that they weigh themselves too often. Our bodies are constantly fluctuating in weight, sometimes by as much as 5 pounds (30). So one morning you might weigh yourself, and the scale may say you lost weight, so you're happy. Then the next day you step on the scale, and now you gained half a pound.

At this point, you'd be freaking out and wondering, "What in the world is going on?" Imagine having to fight this psychological battle each and every week. Every week you have to overcome negative thoughts and worries:

- Is my diet actually working?
- Am I doing something wrong?
- Should I quit?
- Should I try a different nutritional approach?

You would have to overcome all of those doubts before you could start making any real progress. The reality is that nothing is wrong with you; it is the scale that's deceiving you. It's making you think that you've gained weight, when in reality, your bodyweight is simply fluctuating.

Therefore it's important to weigh yourself as consistently as you possibly can. Weigh yourself first thing in the morning before you've eaten anything. In addition to that, only weigh yourself once a week. One week is long enough for you to know if the weight on the scale has gone down it's because of actual weight loss, not because of a fluctuation.

Overall, I want you to focus on the bigger picture when it comes to weight loss. Over the past 3 months, has the direction on the scale been going the way you want it to? If so then great, you're making progress and that's what matters. Don't freak out and question everything you're doing, all because you didn't lose any weight one week.

Chapter 8: What to Do for Exercise

The vegan keto diet is a great nutrition strategy, but you can also use it to help maximize fat loss in the gym. There are a couple of different ways to take advantage of this. The first way is by being glycogen depleted when you workout. All you need to do is workout in the morning or early afternoon before you've eaten anything.

When you workout in a fed state, your body will use the glycogen in your body as fuel for energy. However, when you workout with your body's glycogen stores depleted, your body won't be able to tap into your glycogen stores for energy. It'll have to go somewhere else. Guess where that somewhere else is? Your fat stores!

So by working out in this state, your body will become more efficient at using fat for energy instead of carbs. The second thing you can do to maximize fat loss from working out is delay eating after your workout. The media has done a good job of making us think we must immediately consume protein after a workout or else it was a waste. Research shows that your body won't lose muscle if you don't eat protein within 45 minutes of your workout (31).

Whenever you workout, your body's growth hormone levels will increase (32). This growth hormone will help to protect your muscle and increase fat burning. However if you eat right after you finish a workout, your growth hormone levels will be blunted, and insulin levels will increase. For this reason, you'll want to delay eating anything after finishing a workout for 1-2 hours.

Eating more calories won't help you lose more weight. Yet, when it comes to eating after a workout, people act like they're immune to gaining fat from these extra calories. "I hit it hard in the gym today, I deserve a large milkshake!" No, you don't.

Imagine you go to the gym and burn 300 calories. Then, immediately after your workout, you consume a 350-calorie post workout protein shake. Now you've completely wiped out all of the calories you burned from the workout, plus you ate an additional 50 calories! It's ok to eat a meal after working out if that's when you would normally eat anyway.

Don't go out of your way to eat extra calories for the sake of a post workout shake—it won't help you burn more fat! You might be weary of working out before eating anything if you usually workout in a fed state. Give it a try for 1-2 weeks to give your body a chance to adapt to it. Once you do, you should notice that you have more focus and intensity in the gym.

Here's a good beginner's workout plan you can do if you're unsure of what to do in the gym:

This regimen consists of 3 full-body weight workouts per week. You'll complete the same workout every time you go to the gym. You can set up your workout schedule in one of the following ways:

Monday: Workout
Tuesday: Rest
Wednesday: Workout
Thursday: Rest
Friday: Workout
Saturday: Rest
Sunday: Rest

Or

Monday: Rest
Tuesday: Workout
Wednesday: Rest
Thursday: Workout
Friday: Rest
Saturday: Workout
Sunday: Rest

As a beginner, full-body workouts will provide you with many benefits:

-You'll burn more calories from your workouts.
-You'll gain strength and muscle faster since you'll be stimulating your muscles more frequently.
-You'll have better nervous system recovery because you won't train on consecutive days.
-You'll develop perfect form on key lifts faster because you practice them more often.

Essentially, your body has never been exposed to this stimulus (i.e. weightlifting) before. Therefore, you can take advantage of what some people call "newbie gains." And by increasing the frequency at which you stimulate your muscle groups, you can speed up the process.

Side Note: A set is a group of consecutive repetitions. A repetition is one complete motion of an exercise. And the rest period is how long of a break you'll take until you start the next set. For example, let's say you're completing 3 sets of 8 reps and resting 2 minutes in between sets for the barbell squat exercise.

You'll squat down and stand back up, completing the motion of the exercise and one rep. You'll repeat that motion 7 more times for a total of 8 repetitions. That will complete the set and you will begin your rest period. Once your 2-minute rest period is up, you'll start the next set and perform another 8 repetitions.

That will complete set number 2, and you'll rest another 2 minutes. Once that time period is up, you'll complete the final set of 8 repetitions, and then you'll move onto the next exercise.

Here's the workout:

- Incline Barbell Bench Press: 3 sets 8 reps, 2 min rest between (btw) sets
- Barbell Back Squats: 3 sets of 8 reps, 2 min rest btw sets
- Lat Pulldowns: 3 sets of 10 reps, 90 sec rest btw sets
- Seated DB Military Press: 3 sets of 8 reps, 2 min rest btw sets
- Standing DB Curls: 3 sets of 12 reps, 60 sec rest btw sets
- Tricep Rope Pushdowns: 3 sets of 12 reps, 60 sec rest btw sets

That's all there is to it! Don't let the simplicity of it fool you—it will work.

What About Cardio?

If you're looking to burn fat, cardio can definitely be a handy tool to help you out. It's a great form of exercise you can do, regardless of whether you're into weight training or not. Cardio will do one of two things for you:

#1: Speed up the rate at which you lose fat.
Or

#2: Give you some extra leeway in your diet.

Cardio is by no means necessary for you to reach your fat loss goals, but it will help. What type of cardio should you do—slow and steady or running? Science shows that the best type of cardio you can do is something called high intensity interval training (HIIT) (33).

This kind of cardio combines high intensity cardio with low intensity cardio. HIIT by itself is very effective, but it can be maximized when you immediately follow it with slow steady state cardio. The intensity of the HIIT will release free fatty acids into your bloodstream, and the slow steady state cardio will burn them off. Here's how to perform this hybrid cardio workout:

Part 1: HIIT

Alternate between a high intensity and a low intensity for 10-15 minutes on your choice of cardio machine. Here's an example on a treadmill:
-Run at 7.5 mph for 1 minute
-Walk at 3.5 mph for 1 minute
-Repeat for 10-15 minutes

Part 2: Slow steady state cardio (done immediately after HIIT)

Example on a treadmill: Walk at a constant pace of 3.5-4 mph for 10-15 minutes

Note: If you need to adjust the intensity of the HIIT, then do so. You can alter the run-walk ratios (i.e. run for 30 seconds and walk for 1.5 minutes), or you can decrease the intensity of each run (i.e. run at 6 mph instead of 7.5). And if what I prescribed is too easy, then ramp up the intensity accordingly.

Yes, the vegan keto diet alone will be enough to help you start losing weight and exercise isn't mandatory for it to work. However, exercise will provide you with many additional health benefits and it'll help you lose more weight (34).

Chapter 9: 53 Vegan and Ketogenic Recipes

Note: You can certainly choose to do exclusively the ketogenic or vegan diet and not combine them. If you do want to combine the diets, you may choose to do the cyclical keto diet, in which case your carb intake will be higher. Therefore, not all of these recipes will pertain solely to the standard ketogenic vegan diet. Some of the recipes will be exclusively ketogenic, others exclusively vegan, and some keto vegan. Enjoy!

Vegan Recipes

Vegan Breakfast

Ingredients:

- 1 cup of warm water
- 2 cups of coffee
- 1 tbls coconut oil
- 2 tbls (15 grams) NutriBiotic brown rice vanilla protein powder
- 12 raw almonds

Directions:

1. Using a blender and a deep container that holds at least 2 cups, blend the hot coffee, coconut oil, and brown rice protein powder.
2. Pour this mixture into your coffee cup, and drink this while you eat the 12 almonds.

3. Pour another cup of coffee into the same cup to get the rest of the protein powder that may have stuck to the bottom.

Number of servings: 1

Macros (per serving):

Calories: 282.8
Protein: 15.8 g
Carbs: 7.1 g
Fat: 21.1 g

Vegan Chocolate Ice Cream

Ingredients:

- 1, 15oz can of coconut milk
- 2 tbsp. xylitol
- 2 tbsp. unsweetened cocoa powder
- 1/2 cup unsweetened plain almond milk

Directions:

1. Mix together all ingredients until thoroughly combined.
2. Move the mixture to a container and seal with a lid.
3. Put mixture in freezer for about 2-3 hours, and stir the mixture every half-hour.
4. Serve and enjoy!

Number of servings: 6

Macros (per serving):

Calories: 159.5
Protein: 2.0 g
Carbs: 3.4 g
Fat: 15.8 g

Vegan Coconut Truffles

Ingredients:

- 1 tbsp. raw organic coconut oil
- 1 tbsp. unsweetened shredded coconut
- 1/2 tsp. xylitol
- 1 tbsp. cocoa powder

Directions:

1. Blend together the coconut oil, shredded coconut and xylitol.
2. Refrigerate until set, which should be roughly 10 minutes.
3. Cut into 2 cubes or roll into 2 balls.
4. Next roll the cubes/balls in the cocoa powder.
5. Serve and enjoy!

Number of servings: 2

Macros (per serving):

Calories: 113.8
Protein: 1.0 g
Carbs: 3.2 g
Fat: 11.7 g

Guacamole

Ingredients:

- 4 avocadoes
- 1 tub fresh salsa, pico de gallo style, including vinegar brine
- 3/4 cup chopped fresh cilantro
- 1/4 - 1/2 t salt
- 1/4 t chopped garlic

Directions:

1. Put all of the ingredients in a blender and mix together.
2. Place guacamole in a bowl and cover with wax paper to prevent browning and then seal the bowl.
3. Allow guacamole to sit at least 1 hr before serving.

Number of servings: 16

Macros (per serving):

Calories: 79.1
Protein: 0.8 g
Carbs: 4.7 g
Fat: 6.8 g

Spanish Rice

Ingredients:

- 1/2 head cauliflower, grate in a food processor
- 2 green onions, diced
- 1 tomato, diced
- 1/2 orange bell pepper, diced
- 1/2 jalapeno pepper, diced
- 1-tbsp. fresh lemon juice
- 2 tbsp. cilantro, minced
- 1/2 an avocado, mashed
- 1/2-tsp. chili powder
- 1/2-tsp. paprika
- 3/4 tsp. sea salt

Directions:

1. Grate cauliflower in a food processor.
2. Puree the remaining ingredients together in food processor until it creates a guacamole-like consistency.
3. Add in the grated cauliflower to the mixture, mix, and serve!

Number of servings: 2

Macros (per serving):

Calories: 130.0
Protein: 4.7 g
Carbs: 16.1 g
Fat: 7.4 g

Vegan Energy Bars

Ingredients:

- 1/4-cup sunflower seed butter
- 1/4-cup chia seeds
- 2 tbsp. cacao powder
- 2 tbsp. PB2
- 1 tbsp. coconut butter
- 1/4 cup unsweetened reduced-fat shredded coconut
- 2 tbsp. almond flour

Directions:

1. Add all ingredients together minus the final 1/4-cup shredded coconut.
2. Press the mixture into a small container lined with waxed paper and refrigerate for 1-2 hours to make slicing easier.
3. Once sliced, coat the bars with the final 1/4-cup of shredded coconut.
4. Individually wrap each bar in waxed paper.
5. Store in refrigerator overnight, serve and enjoy!

Number of servings: 4

Macros (per serving):

Calories: 231.1
Protein: 9.6 g
Carbs: 16.0 g
Fat: 16.4 g

Vegan Protein Muffins

Ingredients:

- 30 grams (about 1/4 cup) brown rice protein powder
- 1/4 cup flax meal
- 1/2 tsp. baking powder
- 1/4-tsp. baking soda
- 1/8-tsp. salt
- 1/4-tsp. liquid stevia (more or less)
- 5 tbsp. water
- 1-tsp. rice vinegar

Directions:

1. Preheat oven to 350 degrees F.
2. Grease a round ramekin with palm shortening.
3. In a small bowl, put the protein powder, flax meal, baking powder, baking soda, salt in the bowl and mix together.
4. Next add in and stir in the water, stevia, and vinegar.
5. Spread into the prepared ramekin, making a thick batter.
6. Bake mixture for roughly 20 minutes.
7. Remove from ramekin and let cool briefly before serving.

Number of servings: 2

Macros (per serving):

Calories: 120.6
Protein: 15.0 g
Carbs: 6.3 g
Fat: 4.5 g

Vegan Taco Dinner

Ingredients:

- 2 cups textured vegetable protein
- 2 cups boiling water
- 1/4-cup olive oil
- 1 packet of Publix taco seasoning mix

Directions:

1. Put the textured vegetable protein into a bowl with the seasoning packet.
2. Add in the boiling water and olive oil and mix the ingredients together.
3. Cook over medium heat in a pan sprayed with cooking oil.
4. Cook until lightly browned, serve and enjoy!

Number of servings: 8

Macros (per serving):

Calories: 154.7
Protein: 12.0 g
Carbs: 9.2 g
Fat: 6.8 g

Vegan Peanut Butter Cups

Ingredients:

- 8 oz (8 squares) divided Baker's unsweetened chocolate
- 1-cup chunky natural peanut butter
- 5-pitted Medjool dates
- 1/2-cup divided agave nectar
- 1/4-cup divided unrefined virgin coconut oil

Directions:

1. Line mini muffin tin with mini cupcake liners.
2. Melt 4 oz. (4 squares) of the chocolate in a double boiler over medium heat and stir frequently with a silicon spatula until melted.
3. Add 2 tbsp. of the coconut oil and 3 tbsp. of the agave nectar and mix well, and immediately remove from heat.
4. Use a spoon to spread the chocolate mixture into the bottom of the cupcake liners.
5. Place the peanut butter and dates into a food processor with 2 tbsp. of the agave nectar and blend until well combined.
6. Roll the peanut butter mixture into small, 3/4-inch balls and flatten, and press one into each cup.
7. Repeat step 2 exactly with the other half of the chocolate, oil, and agave nectar.
8. Spread the chocolate mixture on top of the cups, sealing in the peanut butter mixture.
9. Place the tins in the fridge to harden for 2 hours, serve and enjoy!

Number of servings: 24

Macros (per serving):

Calories: 147.9
Protein: 4.0 g
Carbs: 9.7 g
Fat: 12.6 g

Vegan Cauliflower Macaroni and Cheese

Ingredients:

- 2, 1/2 Cups Pre-Grated Cauliflower

Cheese Sauce Ingredients:

- 3 tbsp. ground flax
- 3 tbsp. unsweetened almond milk
- 7 tbsp. nutritional yeast
- 1 tsp. melted coconut oil
- 2 tsp. stone ground mustard
- 1/4 tsp. garlic powder
- 1/4 tsp. onion powder
- 1/4 tsp. sea salt
- 1/2 tsp. Sriracha hot sauce
- Pepper to taste

Topping Ingredients:

- 1 tbsp. almond flour
- 1 tbsp. nutritional yeast

Directions:

1. Preheat oven to 450 degrees F.
2. In a large skillet cook grated cauliflower until translucent, which will be roughly 7-10 minutes on medium heat.
3. In a large bowl put all of the cheese sauce ingredients together and mix well.
4. Add in the cauliflower to the cheese sauce and stir well.
5. Scoop cauliflower into ramekins or a baking dish.
6. Top the mixture with almond flour and nutritional yeast topping.
7. Put the mixture in the oven and bake for about 25-30 minutes or until golden brown

8. Remove from oven, let cool, and enjoy!

Number of servings: 3

Macros (per serving):

Calories: 217.3
Protein: 16.3 g
Carbs: 24.2 g
Fat: 8.5 g

Vegan French Onion Soup

Ingredients:

- 1/2 oz. grams of Earth Balance soy free
- 8 oz. white onions, sliced into thin strips
- 13 oz. of Pacific Organic Vegetable Broth low sodium
- 6 1/2 oz. Water
- 1/2 tsp. thyme
- Salt and pepper to taste

Directions:

1. Add Earth Balance to stovetop pot and melt on medium heat.
2. Once the pot starts to sizzle, add in the thinly sliced onions.
3. Cook under caramelized, or about 15 minutes.
4. Stir constantly under golden brown.
5. Add pepper and thyme and stir, and then add in the broth and water.
6. Bring to a boil, reduce heat to a simmer and cook covered for 5 minutes.
7. Take off heat and rest for another 5 minutes, serve and enjoy!

Number of servings: 4

Macros (per serving):

Calories: 52.1
Protein: 0.6 g
Carbs: 6.0 g
Fat: 2.8 g

Vegan Lentil Soup

Ingredients:

- 2 cups rinsed lentils
- 1 cup grated carrots
- 1 cup chopped celery
- 1 cup chopped onions
- 3 cloves garlic, minced or crushed
- 1 tbs. paprika
- 1 tsp. chili powder
- 2 tsp. salt
- 1 tsp. black pepper
- 6 cups water

Directions:

1. Rinse lentils and cover with 6 cups water in a large pot, or enough to nearly fill the pot.
2. Cook for about half an hour on medium heat.
3. Next, add all the veggies and seasonings.
4. Cook another half hour to hour, or until all veggies and lentils are soft, on medium heat.
5. Serve and enjoy!

Number of servings: 10

Macros (per serving):

Calories: 63.1
Protein: 4.2 g
Carbs: 11.8 g
Fat: 0.4 g

Vegan Stuffed Shells

Ingredients:

Ingredients for the Ricotta

- Tofu, extra firm, 1 block
- Lemon juice from 1/2 lemon
- 1 clove of minced garlic
- 1/4 tsp. salt
- 10 basil leaves
- 2 tsp. olive oil
- 4 tbsp. nutritional yeast

Ingredients for Shells:

- 3 oz. jumbo shells
- 1 1/4 Francesco Rinaldi Tomato & Basil pasta sauce

Directions:

- Preheat oven to 350 degrees F.
- Drain and press the tofu and mush it in a large bowl.
- Add lemon juice, garlic, salt and pepper, and chopped basil to the tofu and mush again.
- Add olive oil, stir with a fork, and add nutritional yeast. Continue mixing all of the ingredients and then cover the bowl and place in the fridge.
- Boil the pasta shells according to box directions and drain the pasta.
- Pour the majority of the spaghetti sauce into a glass 9"x13" baking pan. Take each of the shells and put a spoonful of ricotta in each.
- Sauce the top of the shells and cover the pan with foil.
- Bake for 25 minutes, take the foil off and bake for another 10 minutes.
- Let cool for ten minutes, serve and enjoy!

Number of servings: 10

Macros (per serving):

Calories: 111.1
Protein: 6.2 g
Carbs: 8.1 g
Fat: 5.8 g

Vegan Pumpkin Pancakes

Ingredients:

- 2 1/2 cups whole-wheat flour
- 2 1/2 cups water
- 1/2-cup soymilk
- 2 tbsp. baking powder
- 1 tsp. salt
- 1/2 cup mashed, cooked pumpkin
- 1/2 tsp. cinnamon
- 1/4 tsp. nutmeg
- 1/4 tsp. allspice
- 1 tsp. vanilla extract
- 1/2 tsp. baking soda
- 1 tsp. apple cider vinegar

Directions:

1. Put the soymilk and the tsp. vinegar in a bowl, and give it 5 minutes to curdle.
2. After the 5 minutes, add in and stir together the pumpkin, spices, water and soymilk.
3. Add in remaining ingredients and stir until moist.
4. Let the mixture sit for 5 minutes to rise and then lightly stir again.
5. Let rest 5 more minutes and cook them up into 4" pancakes.

Number of servings: 20

Macros (per serving):

Calories: 59.5
Protein: 2.2 g
Carbs: 13.0 g
Fat: 0.4 g

Vegan Chickpea Casserole

Ingredients:

- 14 oz. can chickpeas
- 1 tbsp. olive oil
- 14 oz. can tomatoes
- 1 large, sliced onion
- 1 tbsp. curry powder
- 2 tbsp. smooth peanut butter
- 1 1/2 oz. of raisins
- 1/2 cup unsweetened apple juice

Directions:

1. Sauté onion in olive oil
2. Add in chickpeas, curry, canned tomatoes, peanut butter, raisins and apple juice
3. Cook for 15 minutes.
4. Serve and enjoy!

Number of servings: 4

Macros (per serving):

Calories: 280.5
Protein: 8.8 g
Carbs: 44.6 g
Fat: 9.1 g

Black-Eyed Peas and Tomatoes

Ingredients:

- 3 tbsp. olive oil
- 1 cup of diced onions
- 3-4 cloves of minced garlic
- 2 (10 oz.) pkg. frozen black eyed-peas
- 1 (16 oz) can of stewed drained tomatoes
- Salt and pepper to taste

Directions:

1. Combine the onions and oil in a small sauté pan, with a lid.
2. Cover and cook the onions over low to low-medium heat for 20-30 minutes, stirring occasionally.
3. Add in the peas and the canned tomatoes, including the tomato liquid.
4. Bring to a boil, cover the pan and simmer on low heat for 20 minutes.
5. The peas should be tender and the sauce should have thickened.
6. Season with salt and pepper, serve, and enjoy!

Number of servings: 4

Macros (per serving):

Calories: 270.6
Protein: 6.0 g
Carbs: 39.3 g
Fat: 10.9 g

Vegan Seitan Fajitas

Ingredients:

- 1 pkg. seitan
- 1 medium chopped onion
- 1 green chopped pepper
- 1/2 cup frozen corn
- 1 tbsp. chili powder
- 1/4-cup water
- 8 corn tortillas
- Salsa to taste

Directions:

1. Cut the seitan into small bite-size pieces and set to the side.
2. Spray a large non-stick skillet with cooking spray.
3. Cook the onion over medium-high heat until soft, and stir occasionally for 5 minutes.
4. Add the corn, green pepper, seitan, chili powder and water to the pan and continue cooking until the peppers are soft.
5. Warm the tortillas and place fajita mixture along with 1 tbsp. of salsa in each tortilla.
6. Serve and enjoy!

Number of servings: 4

Macros (per serving):

Calories: 225.7
Protein: 16.3 g
Carbs: 37.8 g
Fat: 2.8 g

Vegan Carrot and Ginger Soup

Ingredients:

- 1 tbsp. olive oil
- 1-1/2 cups diced onions
- 2-3 cloves of minced garlic
- 4 cups fresh chopped carrots
- 1 to 1-1/2 tsp. of grated ginger
- 4 cups vegetable broth
- 1/4 cup orange juice
- 3 cups rice milk
- Salt and pepper to taste

Directions:

1. Sauté the olive oil, onions and garlic in a large pot for 4 minutes
2. Add in the carrots, ginger, and broth and boil for 30 minutes or until the carrots are tender.
3. Puree the mixture in a food processor.
4. Move the mixture to the stove and heat until warm.
5. Add in the orange juice and rice milk, but don't boil it
6. Add salt and pepper to taste, serve, and enjoy!

Number of servings: 6

Macros (per serving):

Calories: 147.3
Protein: 1.9 g
Carbs: 27.7 g
Fat: 3.6 g

Vegan Salad Pasta

Ingredients:

- 4 cups whole-wheat pasta
- 1/4-cup red wine vinegar
- 1/4-cup balsamic vinegar
- 1 tbsp. dijon mustard
- 1/4-cup extra virgin olive oil
- 2 cloves of minced garlic
- Salt and pepper to taste
- 1/4 cup olives
- 1 small zucchini

Directions:

1. Cook all of the pasta according to package directions and drain it.
2. Drizzle the pasta with half the olive oil to prevent sticking and set aside.
3. Chop olives and zucchini and set them aside.
4. Combine both vinegars, dijon mustard, remaining olive oil, and garlic and whisk them together.
5. Coat pasta with the mixture, and add in zucchini and olives. After that, add salt and pepper to taste.
6. Serve and enjoy!

Number of servings: 4

Macros (per serving):

Calories: 368.8
Protein: 7.9 g
Carbs: 45.5 g
Fat: 18.1 g

Vegan Banana Peanut Butter Smoothie

Ingredients:

1 large frozen banana
4 tbsp. peanut butter
1-cup rice milk
2 tbsp. ground flax seeds

Directions:

1. Put banana, peanut butter, rice milk, and flax seeds in a blender and blend until smooth.
2. Serve and enjoy!

Number of servings: 1

Macros (per serving):

Calories: 684.6
Protein: 21.5 g
Carbs: 73.2 g
Fat: 39.8 g

Vegan Pinto Bean Burger

Ingredients:

- 2 cups of canned pinto beans
- 1/2-cup Salsa
- 2 tbsp. flax seed meal
- 1 tsp. chili powder
- 1/2 tsp. cumin seed
- 4 oz. crushed tortilla chips

Directions:

1. Preheat oven to 350 degrees F.
2. Combine flaxseed meal with 3 tbsp. water; let it sit for one minute until it forms a paste.
3. In a small mixing bowl, combine all ingredients, and mix together until smooth.
4. Form mixture into six patties, and coat both sides with cooking spray.
5. Place patties on a baking sheet, and bake for 20 minutes
6. Serve and enjoy!

Number of servings: 6

Macros (per serving):

Calories: 166.1
Protein: 6.2 g
Carbs: 26.2 g
Fat: 6.5 g

Vegan Spinach Casserole

Ingredients:

- Olive oil for frying
- 1 cup each of chickpeas, pinto, and kidney beans
- 1/2 large onion
- 3 cloves of chopped garlic
- 1 cup of thinly sliced red bell peppers
- 10 pitted and chopped black olives
- 2 tins of tomatoes
- 2 tbsp. tomato puree
- 1/2 tsp. salt
- Dash of soy sauce
- Black pepper to taste
- Fresh basil to taste
- 1 bay leaf

Directions:

1. In a large saucepan add the olive oil and fry the onion then add in the garlic.
2. Toss in the peppers and olives, frying for 5 minutes continuously stirring.
3. Then add in all 3 different kinds of beans.
4. Cook for another 10 minutes, stirring every now and then to make sure the beans don't stick to the bottom of the pan.
5. Add both tins of tomatoes, the tomato paste, salt, soy sauce, and bay leaf and place a lid over the saucepan.
6. Simmer on a low heat for an hour to an hour and a half, stirring roughly every 10 minutes.
7. 10 minutes before cooking time is finished, add some chopped basil to taste.
8. Serve and enjoy!

Number of servings: 6

Macros (per serving):

Calories: 205.1
Protein: 8.2 g
Carbs: 31.6 g
Fat: 6.1 g

Vegan Stuffed Bell Peppers

Ingredients:

- 6 bell peppers
- 1 can (2 cups) of tomato sauce
- 1 large chopped onion
- 2 cups of sliced mushrooms
- 1 bunch of fresh spinach
- 2 cloves of crushed garlic
- 2 tbsp. of fresh basil
- 1 jalapeño pepper
- 1 cup cooked brown rice
- 1/2 cup of shredded tempeh
- Soy sauce to taste

Directions:

1. Preheat oven to 350 degrees F.
2. Chop all the ingredients minus the bell peppers.
3. Place all the ingredients in a large pot and add olive oil, garlic cloves, fresh basil, jalapeño and onions and cook on high heat for 3 minutes.
4. Add the mushrooms and tempeh and simmer on medium heat for 5 minutes.
5. Toss in the spinach and the rice and cover the pan and turn off the heat to help blend the flavors together.
6. Cut the tops off of the peppers and place the tops to the side.
7. With a spoon, scoop out the seeds from the inside of the bell peppers.
8. Fill the peppers with the mixture and place the tops back on them.
9. Put peppers in a lightly oiled casserole dish and place in oven.
10. Bake the peppers for about 15 minutes.
11. Let cool for 5 minutes, serve, and enjoy!

Number of servings: 6

Macros (per serving):

Calories: 160.6
Protein: 8.8 g
Carbs: 29.9 g
Fat: 2.7 g

Vegan Lettuce Wraps

Ingredients:

- 1 large carrot
- 1 spear (5" long) of broccoli
- 1/2 cup of sliced mushrooms
- 1/2 cup of raw chopped onions
- 1/4 head of a small (4" diameter) red cabbage
- 1/2-cup green beans
- 2 tbsp. olive oil
- 2 tbsp. soy sauce
- 4 large leaves of iceberg lettuce

Directions:

1. Chop all of the vegetables.
2. Add 2 tbsp. olive oil to a wok, and turn stove heat on high.
3. Add onions to hot oil and cook for 1 minute.
4. Add remaining vegetables, stir, and cover for 1 minute.
5. Repeat until vegetables have reached desired texture.
6. Add soy sauce, cook 30 seconds longer, while stirring to coat the vegetables with the sauce.
7. Pour into bowl and serve with lettuce leaves.

Number of servings: 2

Macros (per serving):

Calories: 212.2
Protein: 3.6 g
Carbs: 20.4 g
Fat: 14.0 g

Vegan Potato Leek Soup

Ingredients:

- 6 cups vegetable broth
- 7 small, chopped potatoes
- 3 thinly sliced leeks
- 3-4 cloves of garlic
- A splash of almond milk
- Salt and pepper to taste

Directions:

1. Chop up the potatoes and Boil them in a large soup pan with the vegetable broth.
2. Continue to cook potatoes until soft, and then use a potato masher to mash them up.
3. In a frying pan, sauté the garlic and leeks with a couple tbsp. of water.
4. Once they are soft, add them to the soup pan with the broth and potatoes.
5. Add a splash of almond milk, salt, and pepper, and let it all simmer for 10 minutes.

Number of servings: 10

Macros (per serving):

Calories: 120.5
Protein: 3.0 g
Carbs: 27.0 g
Fat: 0.3 g

Vegan Bean and Garden Vegetable Soup

Ingredients:

6 cups of vegetable broth
2 large peeled and diced carrots
1 large diced onion
4 cloves of minced garlic
1/2 head of chopped cabbage
1/2 lb. frozen green beans
2 tbsp. tomato paste
1 1/2 tsp. dried basil and oregano
1 tsp. of salt and pepper
1 large diced zucchini
1, 19oz can of dried and rinsed cannellini beans

Directions:

1. Sauté carrots, onion, and garlic in a large non-stick pot for 5 minutes
2. Add all of the remaining ingredients minus the zucchini and cannellini beans and bring to a boil.
3. Cover, reduce heat to medium and simmer for 15 minutes or until the beans are tender.
4. Add the zucchini and cannellini and cook until the zucchini is tender, which will be roughly 7 minutes

Number of servings: 12

Macros (per serving):

Calories: 75.7
Protein: 3.8 g
Carbs: 15.1 g
Fat: 0.3 g

Vegan Beetroot Salad

Ingredients:

- 4 cubed beetroots
- 1 grated carrot
- 1 cubed green apple
- 3 tbsp. of sunflower seeds
- Squeeze of fresh lemon juice
- 2 tsp. olive oil
- Salt and pepper to taste

Directions:

1. Put all of the ingredients in a large bowl and mix well.
2. Serve and enjoy!

Number of servings: 8

Macros (per serving):

Calories: 44.6
Protein: 0.9 g
Carbs: 6.5 g
Fat: 2.1 g

Vegan Eggplant Lasagna

Ingredients:

- 1 medium eggplant
- Non-stick Olive Oil Spray
- 2 lasagna noodles
- 1 (14 oz.) block of tofu
- 1/4 cup minced garlic
- 3 cups of traditional spaghetti sauce
- 8 oz. soy cheese

Directions:

1. Boil the lasagna noodles until tender.
2. While the noodles are cooking, cut the eggplant into thin slices.
3. Spray each slice of eggplant with non-stick olive oil spray.
4. Place the eggplant slices on pan and broil them until the pieces are tender.
5. While the eggplant is cooking, put the tofu and garlic in a food processor.
6. Put a few tablespoons of spaghetti sauce in a 9" x 13" baking dish.
7. Place the two lasagna noodles in the bottom of the pan.
8. Spread a few more tablespoons of sauce on top of the noodles.
9. Spread some of the tofu mixture on top of the sauce.
10. Sprinkle some soy cheese on the top of the tofu mixture.
11. Layer some of the eggplant on top of the cheese.
12. Repeat the previous 3 steps (8-11) until all of the eggplant has been used.
13. Place the remaining sauce, tofu and cheese on top of the last layer of eggplant.
14. Bake at 350 degrees F until the soy cheese is melted.

15. Cut the lasagna into 12 equal slices.
16. Let cool for 10 minutes, serve, and enjoy!

Number of servings: 12

Macros (per serving):

Calories: 130.5
Protein: 9.8 g
Carbs: 16.3 g
Fat: 4.7 g

Vegan Gumbo with Collard Greens

Ingredients:

- 1 bunch of chopped collard greens
- 1/2 tbsp. of olive oil
- 1 cup of chopped onions
- 1 chopped green bell pepper
- 3/4 cup of sliced celery
- 2 tsp. of minced garlic
- 1 cup of chopped tomatoes
- 1/2 tbsp. of ground thyme
- 3 cubes (makes 6 cups) of low sodium vegetable bouillon
- 6 cups of water
- 1 can (15 oz.) of drained red kidney beans
- 1 tsp. of Tabasco sauce
- Salt and pepper to taste

Directions:

1. Prepare the bouillon by dissolving in boiling water and set it aside.
2. Cook the collard greens in a pot of boiling water for 7 minutes, and drain the pot and set it aside.
3. Spray large pot with non-stick cooking spray. Heat the oil in same pot over medium heat.
4. Add the onion, bell pepper, celery, and garlic to the pot, and cook it covered for 5 minutes, occasionally stirring.
5. Toss in the tomatoes and thyme.
6. Add the bouillon broth, and salt and pepper to taste.
7. Simmer on low heat for 30 minutes, and stir occasionally.
8. Add in the collards, beans, and Tabasco sauce.
9. Taste to adjust the seasoning and cook 10 to 15 minutes longer.
10. Serve and enjoy!

Number of servings: 6

Macros (per serving):

Calories: 147.9
Protein: 8.2 g
Carbs: 23.6 g
Fat: 3.6 g

Vegan Italian Skillet

Ingredients:

- 1/2 tbsp. extra virgin olive oil
- 3 links of sliced Tofurky Italian Sausage
- 1/2 cup of diced onion
- 2 large sliced zucchini squash
- 1 (14.5 oz.) can of diced tomatoes w/ basil, garlic, and oregano

Directions:

1. Brown the sausage slices in the olive oil with the onions over medium high heat. Next, add the zucchini, and sweat it for 2 minutes.
2. Throw in the tomatoes, and cover.
3. Simmer for 15 minutes.
4. Serve and enjoy!

Number of servings: 4

Macros (per serving):

Calories: 276.7
Protein: 23.4 g
Carbs: 20.2 g
Fat: 11.6 g

Vegan Tofu Cubes with BBQ

Ingredients:

- 1 block of tofu
- 1 cup of vegan barbecue sauce
- 1 cup of water
- 2 tbsp. of soy sauce
- 1 tbsp. of hot sauce
- 2 tbsp. of granulated sugar
- 2 tbsp. of olive oil

Directions:

1. Dice tofu into cubes about the size of small cubes.
2. Heat oil in frying pan and add tofu.
3. Sauté the tofu on medium until it turn golden.
4. Toss in the ingredients.
5. Stir in the sauces to the mixture
6. Keep cooking on medium until the sauce has thickened.

Number of servings: 4

Macros (per serving):

Calories: 207.7
Protein: 14.4 g
Carbs: 14.1 g
Fat: 11.6 g

Ketogenic (Non Vegan) Recipes

Lemon Garlic Salmon

Ingredients:

- 2 tablespoons unsalted butter
- 2 teaspoons garlic , minced
- 1 teaspoon lemon pepper
- 2 (4 ounce) salmon fillets
- 1 lemon

Directions:

1. Sprinkle salmon fillets on both sides with lemon pepper.
2. In a large skillet, melt butter over medium high heat.
3. Add in garlic.
4. Put salmon in the pan.
5. Cook for 10 minutes per inch of thickness, or until fish flakes when tested with a fork.
6. Flip fillets halfway through cooking to brown other side.
7. Sprinkle with lemon juice before serving.
8. Serve with lemon wedges and a sprig of parsley and enjoy!

Number of servings: 2

Macros (per serving):

Calories: 258.4
Protein: 23.8 g
Carbs: 5.4 g
Fat: 16.7 g

Lemon Rosemary Grilled Chicken Breast

Ingredients:

- 3 tablespoons extra virgin olive oil
- 3 tablespoons fresh lemon juice
- 3 tablespoons white wine
- 1 tablespoon fresh rosemary, chopped
- 4 boneless, skinless chicken breasts
- Salt and pepper to taste

Directions:

1. In a small baking dish, whisk together olive oil, lemon juice, wine and rosemary. Add chicken and turn to coat.
2. Marinate for 45-60 minutes, turning once.
3. Preheat grill and remove chicken breast, season with salt and pepper.
4. Grill chicken over medium high heat until browned, then flip and cook and brown other side.

Number of servings: 4

Macros (per serving):

Calories: 230.2
Protein: 27.3 g
Carbs: 1.2 g
Fat: 11.6 g

Italian Sausage Stuffed Mushrooms

Ingredients:

- Roughly 40 fresh mushrooms
- 1lb. Ground Italian Sausage
- 8oz. Cream Cheese
- 1 can of Rotel
- 1/2 cup mozzarella cheese

Directions:

1. Brown Sausage.
2. Mix in Rotel & Cream Cheese until saucy.
3. Pull out mushroom stems, and scoop out gills.
4. Put mixture into mushrooms & top with mozzarella cheese.
5. Bake at 300 degrees F for 30 minutes.

Number of servings: 10

Macros (per serving):

Calories: 264.3
Protein: 11.0 g
Carbs: 3.2 g
Fat: 23.2 g

Egg Salad

Ingredients:

- 5 large Hard Boiled Egg
- 2 tbsp Mayonnaise, regular
- 2 tsp Dijon Mustard
- 0.125 tsp McCormick Old Bay Seasoning
- 0.5 tsp Celery seed
- 0.5 tsp Black Pepper, freshly ground

Directions:

1. Chop eggs
2. Add mayo, mustard and seasonings to taste
3. Serve in Romaine lettuce leaves, atop a mixed green salad, or in a scooped out avocado half and enjoy!

Number of servings: 2

Macros (per serving):

Calories: 292.0
Protein: 15.9 g
Carbs: 1.7 g
Fat: 23.4 g

Blue Cheese Steak

Ingredients:

- 3 tbsp crumbled blue cheese
- 1/4 cup chopped parsley
- 2 tsp of black, red, and pink peppercorns, cracked
- 1 beef fillet (12 ounces), cut into 3-ounce steaks

Directions:

1. Preheat the oven to 375 degrees F.
2. In a small bowl, put the blue cheese and parsley and use a wooden spoon to loosely work into a paste. Cover and refrigerate.
3. Place the cracked peppercorns onto a plate. Pat the meat dry and roll in the peppercorns to coat on all sides.
4. Put a cast-iron skillet or heavy-bottomed ovenproof sauté pan over moderately high heat.
5. Once hot, place steaks into the dry pan and sear the top and bottom of each steak, 1 to 2 minutes per side.
6. Place 1 tablespoon of the blue cheese mixture on top of each steak and transfer the pan to the oven. Roast 6 to 7 minutes for rare, 7 to 8 minutes for medium.

Number of servings: 4

Macros (per serving):

Calories: 245.8
Protein: 18.5 g
Carbs: 1.2 g
Fat: 18.2 g

Fish Nuggets

Ingredients:

- 1/2 cup of finely ground pork rinds
- 1/2 cup of parmesan cheese
- salt, pepper, or any other seasonings
- 1 egg
- 1 tbsp heavy cream
- 3 frozen vacuum sealed tilapia fillets
- 2 tbsp of oil

Directions:

1. Thaw the fish by letting the still vacuumed fillets sit in a bowl of hot water for a few minutes.
2. Use a food processor or mortar and pestle to finely ground the pork rinds into a powder.
3. In one bowl, thoroughly combine the pork rind powder with the parmesan and whatever spices you like.
4. In a second bowl, whisk the egg and heavy cream.
5. Cut the thawed fish into nuggets (about 1 inch squares.)
6. Heat a skillet to medium-high heat, and then add enough oil to cover the entire surface to a depth of 1/4 inch.
7. Thoroughly cover the fish in the egg mixture on all sides, then thoroughly cover it in the pork rind/cheese mixture and toss it in the oil.
8. Fry until it's golden brown, (about 2-3 minutes) flipping halfway through.

Number of servings: 3

Macros (per serving):

Calories: 432.7
Protein: 50.6 g

Carbs: 0.9 g
Fat: 24.3 g

Broccoli Cheddar Soup

Ingredients:

- 2 tsp. salt
- 3 cups chicken broth
- 1/2 large onion, chopped
- 3 small-med heads of broccoli, chopped into florets
- 1 avocado, roughly chopped
- 1 cup shredded cheddar cheese
- 3 cups heavy whipping cream

Directions:

1. In a large pot, combine broth, salt, onion, and broccoli, and then bring to a low boil.
2. Lower heat, cover, and simmer for 15 minutes or until the broccoli is nice and soft.
3. Put the ingredients of the pot and the avocado in a big blender of food processor and slightly blend it, or thoroughly puree
4. Return to the pot on medium heat, stir in the cheese and heavy cream, bring it back up to a low boil.
5. Simmer for another 10 minutes or so, stirring regularly and enjoy!

Number of servings: 10

Macros (per serving):

Calories: 347.7
Protein: 5.6 g
Carbs: 7.5 g
Fat: 30.9 g

Cauliflower Crust Pizza

Ingredients:

- Cauliflower, raw, 2 cup
- Mozzarella Cheese, whole milk, 1 cup, shredded
- Alfredo - Classico Four Cheese, 0.25 cup
- Hormel Pepperoni (15 Pepperoni), 1.5 serving
- 1 large egg
- Oregano, ground, 1 tsp
- Onion powder, 1 tsp
- 1/4 tsp garlic salt, 1 serving
- Mozzarella Cheese, whole milk, 1 cup, shredded

Directions:

1. In a large bowl, grate the raw cauliflower with a cheese grater.
2. Cook in the microwave for about 4 min.
3. Add one cup of shredded mozzarella and stir. Add the egg, onion powder, oregano, and mix with cheese for 30 seconds.
4. On a cookie sheet, place parchment paper to cover sheet and spray non-stick cooking spray generously.
5. Put the dough mixture onto the parchment paper and spread it out toward the edges.
6. Bake for about 15-20 minutes at 450 degrees F.
7. Add your toppings and put back in the oven for about 2-3 min on high broil.

Number of servings: 10

Macros (per serving):

Calories: 274.0
Protein: 17.4 g
Carbs: 5.6 g
Fat: 20.2 g

Peanut Butter Cream Cheese Bites

Ingredients:

- 4 oz Cream Cheese (softened)
- 1/4 cup Butter, salted (softened)
- 2 tbsp Bell Plantation PB2
- 2 teaspoons of swerve

Directions:

1. Mix all ingredients in a bowl.
2. Drop by tablespoon onto parchment paper.
3. Refrigerate for 1 hour and enjoy!

Number of servings: 10

Macros (per serving):

Calories: 84.1
Protein: 1.4 g
Carbs: 1.0 g
Fat: 8.7 g

Almond Bread

Ingredients:

- 3/4 cup almond flour
- 1-1/2 tsp baking powder
- 1/4 tsp salt
- 1/4 tsp garlic powder
- 1/4 tsp onion powder
- 5 Tsp Unsalted Butter
- 2 Jumbo Eggs.

Directions:

1. Preheat to 375 degrees F.
2. Mix all of the dry ingredients together.
3. Melt the butter in the microwave for 1 minute.
4. Scramble the eggs.
5. Mix the butter and eggs, and add to the dry ingredients.
6. Pour into muffin top pan and bake for 15 minutes.

Number of servings: 8

Macros (per serving):

Calories: 84.1
Protein: 4.3 g
Carbs: 2.6 g
Fat: 6.8 g

Vanilla and Chocolate Fudgesicle

Ingredients:

- 1 scoop vanilla protein powder
- 4 tsp coconut oil
- 14 oz water
- 14 oz Heavy cream
- 1 scoop chocolate protein powder
- 8 Popsicle molds

Directions:

1. Add vanilla protein powder, 7 oz heavy cream, 7 oz water, and 2 tsp coconut oil to a blender.
2. Blend these items together and place in 4 Popsicle molds.
3. Then add the chocolate protein powder, 7 oz heavy cream, 7 oz water, and 2 tsp coconut oil to the blender and mix together.
4. Pour mixture in remaining 4 Popsicle molds.
5. Refrigerate overnight and enjoy!

Number of servings: 8

Macros (per serving):

Calories: 84.1
Protein: 7.0 g
Carbs: 1.9 g
Fat: 31.4 g

Hot Tuscan Chicken Casserole

Ingredients:

- 2 cups cooked chicken
- 1/4 cooked mashed cauliflower
- 1/2 cup cooked bacon chopped
- 1/3 cup chopped sun dried tomatoes
- 2 Tbsp lemon juice
- 1/2 tsp salt
- 1/4 tsp pepper
- 1 cup mayonnaise
- 2 Tbsp red onions
- 1/2 cup Italian blend cheese

Directions:

1. Preheat oven to 350 degrees F.
2. Cook cauliflower in microwave with 2 tsp water for 10 minutes.
3. Mix all ingredients together minus the chicken, cauliflower and cheese.
4. Add in the chicken and cauliflower to mixture. Spread into a baking dish, and top it off with cheese.
5. Cook for 15 minutes, serve, and enjoy!

Number of servings: 4

Macros (per serving):

Calories: 627.6
Protein: 36.9 g
Carbs: 3.7 g
Fat: 51.5 g

Vanilla Pudding

Ingredients:

- 1 cup heavy cream
- 1 cup whole milk
- 1/4 cup cold water
- 2 tbsp water
- 2 tbsp plain gelatin
- 2 tsp vanilla extract
- drops of Stevia to taste

Directions:

1. In a sauce pan, heat 2tbsp of water until bubbly.
2. Add milk and heavy cream to the hot pan and heat until very warm.
3. Sprinkle gelatin over 1/4 c water and let sit for 5 minutes.
4. Add softened gelatin to warmed milk and stir until dissolved. Turn off the stove.
5. Stir in vanilla extract and stevia.
6. Pour into serving bowls/cups and chill for about 30-45 minutes until set.

Number of servings: 4

Macros (per serving):

Calories: 255.3
Protein: 4.0 g
Carbs: 4.5 g
Fat: 24.0 g

Fudge

Ingredients:

- 1/4c Coconut milk
- 1/2 Tsp Vanilla extract
- 1/2 Tsp Salt
- 1/4c Cocoa Powder
- 1c Coconut Oil
- 5 drops Liquid Stevia

Directions:

- Put the coconut oil and coconut milk together in a medium sized bowl and mix with a hand mixer on high for 6 minutes or until well mixed.
- Place the remaining ingredients in the bowl and stir on low speed until the cocoa is added in well. Increase speed and continue mixing until the ingredients are blended together well.
- Place a sheet of parchment or wax paper along the inside of a loaf pan.
- Place the loaf pan in the freezer for at least 15 minutes, until just set.
- Use the edges of the parchment to pull the fudge out of the pan. Place on a cutting board and remove the parchment paper.
- Use a sharp knife to cut the fudge into squares. Store in an airtight container in the freezer.

Number of servings: 12

Macros (per serving):

Calories: 174.8
Protein: 0.4 g
Carbs: 1.3 g
Fat: 19.8 g

Buffalo Chicken Jalapeno Poppers

Ingredients:

- 500 grams Chicken Thigh Bone removed Skin Eaten
- 6 servings Hormel natural choice cherry wood smoked uncured bacon
- 2 pepper Jalapeno Peppers
- 8 oz Cream Cheese
- 8 servings Cheese - HEB Extra Sharp Cheddar Block Cheese
- 16 tsp Frank's Hot Sauce
- 6 tbsp Duke's Mayonnaise
- 7 Mason jars

Directions:

1. De-bone all chicken thighs and preheat oven to 400F. Season chicken thighs well with salt and pepper, then lay on a cooling rack over a cookie sheet wrapped in foil. Bake chicken thighs for 40 minutes at 400F.
2. Once the chicken has cooked for 20 minutes, start on the filling. Chop 6 servings of bacon into pieces and put into a pan over medium heat.
3. Once bacon is crispy, add jalapenos into the pan.
4. Once jalapenos are soft and cooked, add cream cheese, mayo, and frank's red hot to the pan. Mix together these ingredients and season to taste.
5. Remove chicken from the oven and let it cool slightly. Once cooled, remove the skins from the chicken.
6. Evenly divide chicken into 7 portions and place in bottom of mason jar.
7. Spread cream cheese mixture over each chicken layer, then top with the sharp Cheddar cheese.
8. Bake for 10-15 minutes at 400 degrees F. Broil for 3-5 minutes to finish.

Number of servings: 7

Macros (per serving):

Calories: 482.9
Protein: 37.0 g
Carbs: 2.7 g
Fat: 53.2 g

Chili

Ingredients:

- 2 tbsp Chili powder
- 2 tbsp Cumin seed
- 2 tbsp Garlic powder
- 16 oz Pork, fresh, ground, raw
- 1 can (6 oz) Tomato Paste
- 16 oz lean ground beef
- 2 cup water
- 8 serving Bacon - Farmland Thick Sliced Bacon
- 1 cup Red Onion Raw
- 1 medium green bell pepper
- 2-1/2 cup Rotel

Directions:

1. Cut bacon into 1" squares and cook until crisp. Set aside to drain.
2. Chop onion and green pepper and cook in bacon grease until slightly tender. Set aside.
3. Cook ground beef and pork until done.
4. Add cooked onion and pepper, meat, Rotel, tomato paste, and water in Dutch oven.
5. Bring to a boil and cook 15-20 min to meld flavors.
6. Add bacon before serving and enjoy!

Number of servings: 8

Macros (per serving):

Calories: 431.6
Protein: 25.0 g
Carbs: 12.9 g
Fat: 30.5 g

Bacon Cups

Ingredients:

- 12 slices lower-sodium bacon, halved
- 1lb (16oz) Ground beef, lean
- 4 oz Cream Cheese
- 3/4 cup Colby and Monterey Jack Cheese, shredded
- 1/4 tsp Ground Turmeric
- 1/4 tsp Ground Coriander
- 1/4 tsp Paprika
- 1 tsp Onion powder
- 2 tsp Garlic powder
- Salt and pepper to taste

Directions:

1. Preheat oven to 350 degrees F.
2. Arrange bacon in a lightly greased jumbo muffin pan, with 3-4 pieces per cup.
3. Place the bacon in the oven for approximately 10 minutes or until the edges are crisp
4. Combine the cream cheese and all spices in a bowl until smooth and set to the side.
5. Brown the ground beef in a medium saucepan. When it's almost done, add the cream cheese mixture and simmer until the consistency is the same throughout.
6. Spoon half of the beef mixture into the bacon cups, pressing it firmly into the bottom to hold it tightly.
7. Add half of the shredded cheese on top of the beef.
8. Add the rest of the beef mixture, followed by the rest of the cheese.
9. Bake for an additional 10 minutes or until cheese is golden.
10. Let cool for 5 minutes, serve, and enjoy!

Number of servings: 6

Macros (per serving):

Calories: 391.7
Protein: 22.7 g
Carbs: 2.4 g
Fat: 32.6 g

Lasagna

Ingredients:

- 3 serving Bacon, John Morrell, Hardwood Smoked Bacon (2 slices/17g)
- 1 cup, sliced Zucchini
- 2 medium red peppers
- 2 slice (1 oz) Cheddar Cheese
- 8 slice (1 oz) Monterey Cheese
- 2 Italian tomato Red Ripe Tomatoes

Directions:

1. Preheat oven to 425 degrees F
2. Slice Zucchini and layer the bottom of glass pan
3. Slice Roma tomatoes and layer over the Zucchini
4. Layer Slices Monterey Cheese over tomatoes
5. Cut Bacon in half and layer along pan
6. Slice Peppers lengthwise and place over bacon
7. Cover with shredded cheddar cheese
8. Cover loosely with tin foil
9. Bake 45 minutes
10. Remove tinfoil and broil for 15 minutes
11. Remove from oven and let stand 10 minutes
12. Serve and enjoy!

Number of servings: 6

Macros (per serving):

Calories: 270.3
Protein: 15.0 g
Carbs: 10.2 g
Fat: 19.4 g

Gnocchi

Ingredients:

- 150 grams mozzarella cheese, part skim milk
- 2 teaspoons Parmesan cheese
- 2 large egg yolks

Directions:

1. Melt Parmesan and mozzarella cheese in microwave and mix with any seasonings.
2. Add in egg yolks and mix completely
3. Put in fridge for 10 minutes.
4. Bring a pot of water to a boil.
5. Remove dough from fridge and place on parchment paper, and divide dough into 3 pieces.
6. Roll out each dough ball into a strand around 12 inches long and shape it like a long, fat cylinder.
7. Cut into 1-inch pieces and place in boiling water.
8. When they rise to the top, fry them in a pan to make the edges crispy.
9. Serve and enjoy!

Number of servings: 2

Macros (per serving):

Calories: 255.5
Protein: 21.9 g
Carbs: 2.7 g
Fat: 17.2 g

Cauliflower Casserole

Ingredients:

- 1 head, medium (5-6" dia) Cauliflower, raw
- 4 oz Cream Cheese
- 4 tbsp Parmesan Cheese, shredded
- 1/2 cup Sour Cream
- 3 serving Bacon, John Morrell, Hardwood Smoked Bacon (2 slices/17g)
- 4 serving Green Onion (fresh-1 stalk)
- 1 cup, shredded Cheddar Cheese
- 1 tsp Garlic powder

Directions:

1. Preheat oven to 350 degrees F.
2. Cut cauliflower in small prices and fry bacon.
3. Boil cauliflower to soften it.
4. Mix cream cheese, Parmesan cheese, sour cream, bacon, onions, and garlic powder together.
5. When cauliflower is drained, place on top of cream cheese mixture, and mash it like you would potatoes.
6. Put in 8x8 baking dish. Put cheddar on top and 2 slices of crushed bacon.
7. Cook in oven for 20 minutes.
8. Serve and enjoy!

Number of servings: 9

Macros (per serving):

Calories: 181.8
Protein: 8.0 g
Carbs: 5.3 g
Fat: 14.9 g

Tuna Salad

Ingredients:

- 2 (5-oz) cans of tuna
- 2/3-cup Celery, raw, minced
- 2 Tbsp. Sweet Onion, minced
- 1-1/2 Tbsp. Pimiento, (from jar, diced)
- 1/4-cup dill pickle relish
- 1/2-cup mayonnaise
- 3/4 small very ripe avocado
- 2 Eggs, hard-boiled and finely chopped

Directions:

1. Mash ripe avocado and mayonnaise together.
2. Place all ingredients in large bowl and blend thoroughly.
3. Chill before serving and enjoy!

Number of servings: 4

Macros (per serving):

Calories: 338.4
Protein: 17.3 g
Carbs: 5.5 g
Fat: 26.7 g

Swiss Chicken Bake

Ingredients:

- 4 slice (1 oz) Swiss cheese
- 16 oz Tyson boneless, skinless chicken breast
- 8 tbsp mayonnaise
- 8 tbsp HyVee sour cream
- 36 tsp HyVee Parmesan & Romano - 45 serv/container

Directions:

1. Preheat oven to 375 degrees F.
2. Pat chicken dry and put in a greased 9x13 pan.
3. Add sliced cheese on top of chicken breasts.
4. In a bowl blend together mayonnaise, sour cream, 2/3 of the Parmesan cheese, salt, pepper and garlic powder.
5. Spread this over chicken and add remaining Parmesan cheese on top.
6. Bake for 40-50 minutes.
7. Serve and enjoy!

Number of servings: 4

Macros (per serving):

Calories: 576.6
Protein: 43.1 g
Carbs: 2.0 g
Fat: 43.5 g

Chapter 10: Frequently Asked Questions

Do I have to do both the vegan diet and the keto diet at the same time?

No, you certainly don't have to combine the diets and do them both at the same time if you don't want to. You can still get great results from doing only the vegan diet or only the ketogenic diet by itself. The main thing you need to focus on is burning off more calories than you consume. If only following one of the two diets at a time makes things easier for you to follow through, then by all means do it.

How much weight should I lift during the workouts?

Lift as much weight as you possibly can for the given rep range. Initially, you won't know how much weight to use so you'll have to take your best guess. For example, let's say you're doing bench press for 8 reps. You think you can lift around 150 pounds for that many reps, but on your first set you easily complete 10 reps.

This means the weight is too light, and you need to increase it for the next set. On the next set you lift 165 pounds, and you struggle to complete the 8th rep. This is what you want to happen, and it means you've found a good weight to use. Once you can complete all 3 sets for 8 reps with 165 pounds, move up to 170 the next time you bench press. If you can't complete 8 reps for all 3 sets stick with 165 until you can. Here's an example:

Workout 1: Bench Press with 165 pounds
Set 1: 8 reps
Set 2: 8 reps
Set 3: 7 reps

Because you only completed 7 reps on the last set, stick with 165 for the next workout—

Workout 2: Bench Press with 165 pounds
Set 1: 8 reps
Set 2: 8 reps
Set 3: 8 reps

Because you completed all 3 sets for 8 reps move up to 170 on your next workout with bench press.

Note: It's better to use a weight that's too heavy and miss a rep or two than it is to use a weight that's too light and leave some reps in the tank. For example, it's better to do 170 pounds and only complete 6 reps instead of 8 opposed to using 155 pounds and stopping at 8 reps even though you could've easily done more reps.

How Fast Should I Lose Weight?

The more weight you have to lose, the faster the rate at which you can lose the weight. For example, if you have 50+ pounds to lose, you can lose weight at a rate of 2 pounds or more per week. If you only have 5 pounds to lose, then lose weight at a rate of .5 pound per week.

For most people, losing 1 pound per week is the sweet spot. You'll be creating an average caloric deficit of 500 calories daily. At this pace, you'll be losing weight fairly quickly, and you won't be miserable all of the time from a complete lack of calories.

How much water should I drink on a daily basis?

Your body is made up of about 60% water, so it's important to consume water for several reasons:

- It'll help keep your joints and ligaments fluid, which can help prevent injury.

- Water can help control your caloric intake.
- Flush out toxins
- Improve skin quality
- Improve kidney function
- Improve your focus

Many people recommend that you should drink 1 gallon of water per day. This is a blanket answer that doesn't meet individual needs. This recommendation would have a 100-pound woman drinking the same amount of water as a 200-pound man. Absurd!

Other health experts advise drinking eight 8-ounce glasses (64 ounces total) of water a day. But again 64 ounces isn't going to be enough for most people. What should you do then? I don't keep track of my water intake—I go by how I feel and the color of my urine.

Your body's own thirst mechanism will be accurate in telling you if you need more water. If you feel thirsty, then go drink some water. If not, then you're probably ok. You can also use the color of your urine to judge how hydrated you are. If your urine is yellow, then you should drink more water. If it's clear, then you should be good to go. This keeps things simple and it's one less thing you have to keep track of.

How Do I Motivate Myself to Go to the Gym and Eat Healthy?

Finding the motivation to go to the gym or eat right can be hard. No matter who you are, there will be times when you don't feel like working out. Having that feeling is ok, but you can't let it control you. There will be times when you'll have to do it anyway, even when you don't feel like it.

That's what will ultimately separate a long-term successful fitness journey from failing at it. I do have some tips to help you out along the way however:

Tip #1: Focus on Gradual Improvements

Many people make fitness an all-or-nothing game. They tell themselves that they'll workout 5 days a week and eat clean 100% of the time for the rest of their lives. Let's say you workout only 4 days one week. Are you a failure?

Of course not. You still worked out 4 days, but in your mind you are because you failed to reach 5 workouts. You make it hard to celebrate any small successes that you do have because the standards are too high.

Instead, focus on making smaller, more gradual improvements, and celebrate any successes you have along the way. For example, start off with a goal to only workout 2 days per week if it's been years since you've last worked out. Once you achieve that goal, you'll feel good about yourself, and you can move up to working out 3 days per week and so on.

Tip #2: Action Leads Motivation

People think they have to get the inspiration or motivation from somewhere in order to take the action necessary to workout. The reverse of that is actually true. You need to start by taking an action no matter how small. And once you get started, you'll likely want to continue on with what you're doing.

When I think about everything I have to do to workout—put my gym clothes on, drive to the gym, workout with a bunch of grueling exercises, drive back, and shower—I start to make up silly excuses as to why I should skip this time. Instead, I'll tell myself to do just one exercise when I get to the gym. I won't pressure myself to do anything more. After I finish that first exercise, it's always easier for me to finish the rest of the workout.

You just have to get started. Try this out for any healthy habit you want to start. For example, if you want to start flossing your teeth, tell yourself you'll only floss one tooth, and don't pressure yourself to do anything more than that!

Tip #3: Put Your Own Money on the Line

Money is a very powerful motivator. And you can use your own money to motivate yourself to start working out more. Here's what you're going to do—give someone a good amount of money. Not $20, but something that would actually hurt you—$100, $200, $500, or whatever you can't afford to lose.

Then tell your friend that if you don't go to the gym 3 days this week for example, they get to keep the money. When you give up the money in the first place, you'll fight to get it back. This is much different than telling yourself you'll give the money to someone after you miss your workouts.

It's too easy to make an excuse and not give away the money. Give the money up in the first place, and make sure your friend actually holds you accountable to it. This is by far the best way to get motivation to workout. There's a real cost involved if you don't comply. You'll either get ripped or go broke trying.

Conclusion

Thanks for reading this book all the way to the end! I firmly believe that it's truly possible for you to achieve a healthy and good-looking body that you're proud of by following the nutritional and training advice outlined in this book. Getting fit isn't easy, but it's worth it. Stay strong and persist, even when you mess up; you'll succeed in the long run.

Finally, if you have any questions please be sure to email me at thomas@rohmerfitness.com. I'd be more than happy to answer any questions that you have!

Sources

(1) https://www.niddk.nih.gov/health-information/health-statistics/overweight-obesity

(2) https://www.cdc.gov/heartdisease/facts.htm

(3) https://www.ncbi.nlm.nih.gov/pmc/articles/PMC1204764/

(4) https://www.ncbi.nlm.nih.gov/pubmed/8116550

(5) https://www.ncbi.nlm.nih.gov/pubmed/15148063

(6) https://www.ncbi.nlm.nih.gov/pmc/articles/PMC4125607/

(7) https://www.ncbi.nlm.nih.gov/pmc/articles/PMC333231/

(8) https://www.ncbi.nlm.nih.gov/pubmed/15767618

(9) https://www.ncbi.nlm.nih.gov/pubmed/22905670

(10) https://www.ncbi.nlm.nih.gov/pubmed/17313687

(11) http://ajcn.nutrition.org/content/77/5/1146.short

(12) https://www.ncbi.nlm.nih.gov/pubmed/16409560

(13) https://www.ncbi.nlm.nih.gov/pubmed/12088525

(14) http://ajprenal.physiology.org/content/293/4/F974

(15) https://www.ncbi.nlm.nih.gov/pubmed/17228046

(16) http://news.gallup.com/poll/156215/consider-themselves-vegetarians.aspx

(17) https://www.ncbi.nlm.nih.gov/pubmed/24687909

(18) https://www.ncbi.nlm.nih.gov/pubmed/24871675

(19) https://www.cdc.gov/heartdisease/facts.htm

(20) https://www.epa.gov/ghgemissions/sources-greenhouse-gas-emissions

(21) http://usda.mannlib.cornell.edu/usda/nass/LiveSlau//2010s/2017/LiveSlau-08-24-2017.pdf

(22) https://www.cdc.gov/cancer/dcpc/data/types.htm

(23) https://www.cdc.gov/bloodpressure/faqs.htm

(24) https://www.ncbi.nlm.nih.gov/pubmed/25592014

(25) https://www.webmd.com/heart/metabolic-syndrome/metabolic-syndrome-what-is-it#1

(26) https://www.arthritisresearchuk.org/arthritis-information/conditions/osteoporosis/who-gets-it.aspx

(27) https://www.ncbi.nlm.nih.gov/pubmed/11600749

(28) https://www.ncbi.nlm.nih.gov/pubmed/26024494

(29) https://www.ncbi.nlm.nih.gov/pubmed/22825659

(30) https://www.ncbi.nlm.nih.gov/pubmed/23521346

(31) https://www.ncbi.nlm.nih.gov/pubmed/22460474

(32) https://www.ncbi.nlm.nih.gov/pubmed/2796409

(33) https://www.ncbi.nlm.nih.gov/pubmed/8028502

(34) https://www.ncbi.nlm.nih.gov/pmc/articles/PMC1402378/

*Recipes courtesy of users at sparkrecipes.com

Carb Cycling

The Simple Way to Work With Your Body to Burn Fat & Build Muscle

Thomas Rohmer

Copyright © 2018

Rohmerfitness All rights reserved.

No part of this publication may be reproduced, distributed, or
transmitted in any form or by any means, including photocopying, recording, or other electronic or mechanical methods, without the prior written permission and consent of the publisher, except in the in the case of brief quotations embodied in product reviews and certain other non-commercial uses permitted by copyright law.

Disclaimer:

This guide has been created for informational and reference purposes only. The author, publisher, and any other affiliated parties cannot be held in any way accountable for any personal injuries or damage allegedly resulting from the information contained herein, or from any misuse of such guidance. Although strict measures have been taken to provide accurate information, the parties involved with the creation and publication of this guide take no responsibility for any issues that many arise from alleged discrepancies contained herein. It is strongly recommended that you consult a physician, personal trainer, and nutritionist prior to commencing this or any other workout or diet plan. This guide is not a substitute for professional personal guidance from a qualified medical professional. If you feel pain or discomfort at any point during exercises contained herein, cease the activity immediately and seek medical guidance.

Table of Contents

Chapter 1: Not All Carbs Are Created Equally.......131
Chapter 2: The Science Behind How Carb Cycling Works..137
Chapter 3: How to Set Up Your Own Carb Cycling Diet..140
Chapter 4: Macro Percentages for High and Low Carb Days..144
Chapter 5: Carb Cycling and Building Muscle......150
Chapter 6: Muscle Building Workout With Carb Cycling..158
Chapter 7: What About Cardio?..........................164
Chapter 8: 30 Low-Carb Recipes.........................169
Chapter 9: 15 High-Carb Recipes........................204
Chapter 10: How to Track Your Calories and Macros..224
Chapter 11: Frequently Asked Questions..............227

Introduction:

Dieting is hard. Millions of people go on a diet every year, but most will fail to successfully lose weight and keep it off. And it makes sense as to why so few people are successful when trying to get fit. See if you can relate to a story similar to this:

1. You start a new diet.
2. Everything is smooth sailing for the first few weeks and you lose some weight.
3. Eventually, your metabolism slows down, and weight loss comes to a grinding halt.
4. In a desperate attempt to get back on track, you further restrict your calories.
5. You start to go insane because you're eating too few calories.
6. You quit, binge eat, and feel guilty about yourself for quitting.
7. A week or two later, after you've gotten over your latest incident, you decide to go at it again, and the vicious cycle repeats itself.

Luckily, there's a way you can escape this diet trap, and it's called carb cycling. Think of it this way—to get from point A to point B when driving a car, you'll need to use multiple tools: the steering wheel, gas pedal, brakes, etc. to get where you want to go. Most diets only use the gas pedal. It's go, go, go all of the time until you crash and burn.

It's insane to think you'll get anywhere only using the gas pedal of a car! However, with carb cycling, you'll strategically learn how and when to hit the brakes. This'll give your body a chance to recuperate and even further accelerate fat loss!

If that's something you're interested in then you're in the right place. This book will teach you everything you need to know about carb cycling: the science behind it, how to start your own carb cycling diet, and low carb/high carb recipes. Let's jump right in...

Chapter 1: Not All Carbs Are Created Equally

It's first important to understand exactly what carbs are and what their functions are in the body before we get into the ins and outs of carb cycling. Of the three macronutrients: protein, carbs and fat—carbohydrates are your body's first source of energy. Your body will burn off carbohydrates when you exercise to give you the necessary energy to complete the workout. They're also important for serotonin levels in the brain and proper nervous system functioning (1).

Without carbs, your body will soon start to run out of energy and you'll become irritable. If you've ever gone on a low carb diet, you've probably experienced this. For that reason alone, I don't advise going on a low carb diet as a long-term weight loss solution. To clarify, carb cycling isn't a low carb diet.

With carb cycling, you'll strategically have high and low carb days to change things up for continual fat loss. But don't worry about that now, I'll thoroughly explain everything about carb cycling in later chapters. For right now, you need to understand carbs and the differences between simple and complex carbs.

Is a Carbohydrate a Carbohydrate?

Many people love to debate about whether or not a calorie is a calorie. If I eat 100 calories from a cookie and you eat 100 calories from vegetables, are we equal? Well kinda.

One calorie *is* one calorie regardless of what source the calorie came from. Trying to argue with this is like saying one yard of wood isn't the same length as one yard of metal. The difference lies in the *macronutrient* quality.

100 calories from vegetables and 100 calories from a cookie are still 100 calories. Both are made up mostly of carbs; the quality of those carbs is what makes them very different. The cookie contains simple carbs and sugar.

It won't provide you with any vitamins, nutrients, or fiber. It also won't be very satiating. The vegetables, on the other hand, are complex carbs.

They'll provide you with quality complex carbs and a good source of vitamins, nutrients and fiber. Additionally, nutritious foods like fruits and vegetables will keep you fuller longer, which is critical during calorie restriction for weight loss purposes. Therefore, quality of calories can be as important as quantity of calories.

As you can tell, if you eat a low amount of carbs, but the quality of those carbs are poor in nutritional value then you'll still fail. You must eat the right kind of carbohydrates and in the right amounts in order to be successful.

Difference between Simple and Complex Carbohydrates

Many people define simple carbohydrates as carbs that contain sugar and complex carbohydrates as carbs that contain starch and fiber. However, this isn't fully true. Fruit contains sugar, but it's not a simple carbohydrate because it's natural sugar has a different effect on the body than added sugar contained in sodas and processed foods. Not only that, but some starch foods contain refined wheat flour and could cause health issues.

Here's a better way to define complex and simple carbohydrates:

Simple carbs: starches and sugars that have been refined and stripped of their natural nutrients and fiber.

Complex carbs: carbs found in whole, unprocessed foods such as fruits, vegetables, legumes and whole grains.

The main difference between complex and simple carbs is that complex carbs are nutrient dense; this means they contain a large amount of nutrients in relation to the total number of calories they provide. These carbs are rich in fiber, vitamins, minerals and antioxidants. Simple carbs, on the other hand, contain empty calories. They provide little to no nutritional value. Sure they may taste good, but they'll do little to keep you full, which is critical when your calories are restricted.

Health Benefits of Complex Carbs

Eating complex carbs can provide you with the following health benefits:

Fewer Blood Sugar Spikes:

Complex carbs take a longer time to digest, which means that your blood sugar won't spike like it would when you consume simple carbs. When your blood sugar levels increase, your body will release more insulin to digest the incoming carbs. This then leads to a blood sugar crash, which will leave you hungry and craving additional sugar (2).

Potential Reduction in Risk of Developing Chronic Diseases

Antioxidants, fiber, vitamins and minerals are all necessary for preventing disease. By consuming complex carbohydrates, you'll get an adequate dose of all of these, which can reduce you risk for developing certain diseases like diabetes and heart disease (3).

Healthier Digestive Track

Complex carbs contain more beneficial bacteria in them than simple carbs do. This bacteria will help digestive issues from occurring in your gut (4).

Inflammation Reduction:

Long-term inflammation can increase the risk for developing severe diseases. Simple carbs stimulate inflammation, while complex carbs work to reduce inflammation in the body (5).

Dangers of Simple Carbs:

Eating too many simple carbs can be harmful to your health over time. Here are some of the hazards of simple carbs:

They're Easy to Overeat:

Simple carbs are empty calories, which means that they won't satiate you. This'll make it easier to overeat on other foods so you can get full from your meal.

Increased Risk of Disease:

People who consume more sugar and processed foods are more likely to develop heart disease and type 2 diabetes than those who don't (6).

Sugar is Addicting:

There's research to show how addicting sugar can be. Some studies show that sugar can be just as addictive as drugs like cocaine because both cause the brain to release dopamine and stimulate the pleasure centers of our brains (7).

List of High Quality Complex Carbs to Consume in Your Diet

The following is a non-comprehensive list of complex carbs that you should consider eating in your diet on a regular basis:

- Whole Grain Oats
- Quinoa
- Brown rice
- Whole grain barley
- Black beans
- Kidney beans
- Black-eyed peas
- Sweet potatoes
- Chia seeds
- Flax seeds
- Any fruits
- Any green vegetables

List of Simple Carbs to Avoid or Eat Sparingly

The following is a non-comprehensive list of simple carbs that you should avoid eating or only eat in moderation:

- Sodas or beverages that contain excess calories or sugar
- Sweets and pastries such as cake, ice cream, candy, donuts, pop-tarts, etc.
- White bread
- White pastas

Hopefully you now understand the difference between simple and complex carbohydrates, and you can now clearly see that not all carbs are the same. My goal isn't to scare you into never eating any more refined carbs, but I want you to realize the importance of complex carbs. They're going to be critical for your success with carb cycling.

Chapter 2: The Science Behind How Carb Cycling Works

As I mentioned earlier, most diets fail because they only know how to hit the gas pedal and go, go, go. With carb cycling, you're going to go, go, and then hit the breaks and slow down for a bit before putting your foot back on the gas pedal.

When you restrict your caloric intake for a prolonged period of time to lose weight, your leptin levels will decrease. And as you're about to find out, this is a very important hormone for fat loss.

What is Leptin and Why Does it Matter?

Leptin is commonly referred to as the starvation hormone because its main job in the body is to regulate energy balance. At optimal levels, it tells the brain that we have enough fat stored, that we can stop eating and that we can continue burning calories at a normal pace. Essentially, leptin is there to prevent us from starving or overeating. In the hunter and gatherer days, this mechanism was essential for our survival.

Back then, calories were scarce and people didn't know when or where their next meal would come from. During times of food scarcity, leptin would kick in and slow down the person's metabolism and hold onto any fat stores that it could so they could be used at a later time. Fast-forward to the present day and things are much different.

Today, we live in a world with an overabundance of food. You can easily drive to the supermarket or a fast-food restaurant and get food 24/7. Although leptin was necessary for humans to survive this long, it can kind of be a pain-in-the-neck today. Consciously, you know you have access to food whenever you want it, but your body is still in the dark. That's why when you've got your diet down and things are going great, leptin will come in to crash the party. It still thinks you're starving and that food supply is low.

This is how leptin works in the body:

1. We eat
2. Body fat increases
3. Leptin levels increase
4. We eat less and burn more

Or:

1. We don't eat
2. Body fat decreases
3. Leptin levels decrease
4. We eat more and burn less

This is a classic case of "damned if you do, damned if you don't." On one hand, you can eat less, but as soon as you do, your leptin levels will decrease and you'll feel hungry, your appetite will increase and your motivation to exercise will decrease. On the other hand, you can eat more, which will decrease hunger, decrease appetite and increase motivation to workout. Unfortunately though, you're eating more and that's counterproductive to losing weight.

Break the Cycle With Another Cycle

The perfect solution to this catch-22 as you can probably guess is carb cycling. On your low-carb days, your body will be releasing low amounts of insulin, which will allow you to burn more fat. This is because your body doesn't burn off fat when your insulin levels are high; it'll be too busy burning off carbs instead. Of course, having low-carb days will start to decrease your leptin levels.

That's why you'll then have a high-carb day to offset the lowered leptin levels and get them back to normal. Once they're reset, you'll go back to your low-carb days and start burning fat again. You'll change things up at the right moment to trick your body and keep it guessing. You'll never give it the chance to catch onto what you're doing.

The high-carb days will also be beneficial for preserving your body's lean muscle mass. This is true for a couple of reasons:

1. Your glycogen stores will be replenished on your high-carbs, which will help keep your muscle cells full.

2. Your body is more likely to use muscle mass for energy when calories are restricted for extended periods of time (8).

Not only that, but cycling in high carb days will help you keep your sanity and allow you to sustain the diet. When things get hard, we give up and quit. It's much easier to keep going if you know that you're one day away from getting to consume a high amount of carbs again. However, with most diets, you have nothing to look forward to except for more misery. This is what makes having nothing but low-carb days tough, and that's why most people fail with a typical low-carb diet.

Now that you understand how carb cycling is effective, let's get started setting up your own carb cycling diet...

Chapter 3: How to Set Up Your Own Carb Cycling Diet

There are many different ways to set up a carb cycling diet. However, this is the most effective way to go about it:

Monday: Low-carb day
Tuesday: Low-carb day
Wednesday: Low-carb day
Thursday: High-carb day
Friday: Low-carb day
Saturday: Low-carb day
Sunday: Low-carb day
Following Monday: High-carb day

Essentially, you'll have 3 low-carb days in a row and then follow it with a high-carb day. Of course, you don't have to set up your schedule exactly like the example above. You could start your schedule out to where you have a high-carb day on a Saturday for example.

You can also change things around a bit to be more flexible with your schedule so that you eat high-carbs on a day you actually want to. For example, you might have 2 low-carb days in a row, have a high-carb day, and then go 4 days in a row eating a low amount of carbs. You want to have some wiggle room with the diet to make it easier to stick to.

And here's the step-by-step process you need to take to complete your carb cycling diet:

Step #1: Determine Your Total Daily Energy Expenditure (TDEE)

Your TDEE is simply the total number of calories you burn off in a given day. Figuring out your TDEE is the first and most important step in setting up your carb cycling diet. If you don't know your TDEE, you'll be guessing and hoping that you see results. You'll have no idea if you're overeating or eating too few calories.

And in case you're not aware, the following is how your body works in regards to weight loss/gain.

- If you eat more calories than your TDEE, you will gain weight.
- If you eat less calories than your TDEE, you will lose weight.
- If you eat right at your TDEE, then you will neither gain nor lose weight.

Since we're interested in losing weight, we're going to want to eat less than our TDEE. So how do you figure out your TDEE? There are many different equations to determine your TDEE. Regardless of what method you use to find your TDEE, it'll likely be off by 100-200 calories.

For an exact, accurate number, you would have to go to a lab and pay for a test to get it measured. Fortunately, you don't have to waste your time or money doing that. The formulas will be close enough for you to get results. I keep things simple, and this is the formula you'll use to determine your TDEE:

Bodyweight (in pounds) x 13=TDEE

Using myself as an example:

Bodyweight 200 pounds x 13= 2,600 calories

This means:

If I eat more than 2,600 calories per day, I'll start to gain weight.
If I eat less than 2,600 calories per day, I'll start to lose weight.
If I eat 2,600 calories per day, I'll neither gain nor lose weight.

It's pretty simple, right? Sadly, most people have no clue how many calories they're burning off in a given day. And they don't know that they need to eat below their TDEE to start losing weight. They'll blindly start eating healthy and hope for the best. By learning this information, you put yourself ahead of 95% of people who are looking to lose weight.

Step #2: Set Up Your Macros for Low-Carb Days

Carbs are going to make up 20% of your total calories on low-carb days. Full details will be provided for setting up your macros in chapter 4.

Step #3: Set Up Your Macros for High-Carb Days

Carbs will make-up 50% of your total calories on high-carb days. Again, refer to chapter 4 for full details on setting up your macro percentages.

Step #4: Accurately Track and Record Your Calories and Macros

With carb cycling, you want to be as precise as possible with your caloric intake. You can't guess at how many calories certain foods contain. What gets measured gets managed, and in chapter 10, I'll share with you how you can easily and precisely track your calories and macros.

Step #5: Monitor and Adjust Accordingly

Along the way, you might find that you were measuring something wrong or you need to change something. With this step, you'll only make adjustments when necessary. For example, if you go two weeks in a row without losing weight, you'll need to assess and identify what's getting miscalculated so it can be fixed.

Chapter 4: Macro Percentages for High and Low Carb Days

If you're unaware, a macro is short for macronutrient, and they're basically nutrients that provide the body with energy. The body then uses this energy to carry out all of its processes: breathing, organ function, digestion, moving and a whole lot more. There are three macronutrients: protein, carbohydrates and fat. All three macronutrients have their own importance and are essential for survival.

Protein is the body's building block for things like muscle, hair, bones and skin. Fat acts as an insulator for the body, helps maintain normal body temperature and it's used as an energy source when carb stores are low. And as I mentioned earlier, carbs are your body's first source of energy, and they're important for serotonin levels in the brain and proper nervous system functioning.

Macronutrients shouldn't be confused with micronutrients. Micronutrients are nutrients needed in trace amounts for normal growth and development in living organisms. They include things such as vitamins and minerals. However, our main concern with this chapter will be focused on macronutrients. Specifically, the amounts of each macro needed to reach our fitness goals. Before we get into the specific macro percentages, it's important to know the following:

- 1 gram of protein contains 4 calories
- 1 gram of carbohydrate contains 4 calories
- 1 gram of fat contains 9 calories

Knowing this information will help you track the total amount of calories you're consuming for each macronutrient.

Macronutrients for Low-Carb Days

Consume the following macros and calories during your low-carb days:

- **Total calories:** Consume 25% less calories than your total daily energy expenditure (TDEE)
- **Protein:** 1 gram per pound of bodyweight
- **Carbs:** 20% of total calories
- **Fat:** Remaining calories after protein and carbs

I'll use myself as an example for determining the calculations:

As a reminder, calculate your TDEE by multiplying your bodyweight by 13.

Bodyweight=200 x 13= TDEE of 2,600 calories

TDEE on low-carb days:

2,600 x .25= 650

2,600-650=1,950 total daily calories on low-carb days

Protein on low-carb days:

Your protein intake on low-carb days will simply be 1 gram of protein per pound of bodyweight:

1 gram per pound of bodyweight= 200 daily grams of protein

4 calories in 1 gram of protein x 200= 800 total calories from protein

Carbs on low-carb days:

To determine your carb intake on low-carb days, take your TDEE on low-carb days and multiply it by .2:

1,950 x .2= 390 total calories from carbs

You can then divide that number by 4 to get the gram equivalent:

390/4= 97.5 grams of carbs per day

Fat on low-carb days:

Your remaining calories will come from fat. Take your calculated TDEE, subtract your protein and carb calories from that number, and you'll be left with your calories from fat:

1,950 (TDEE)-800 (protein)-390 (carbs)=760 total calories from fat

You can then divide this number by 9 to get the gram equivalent:

760/9= 84.4 grams of fat per day

In summary, this would be my macros and calories on a low-carb day:

TDEE=1,950 calories
Protein= 200 grams (800 calories)
Carbs= 97.5 grams (390 calories)
Fat= 84.4 grams (760 calories)

Macronutrients for High-Carb Days

Consume the following macros and calories on your high-carb days:

- Total calories: Consume 10% less calories than your total daily energy expenditure.
- Protein: 1 gram per pound of bodyweight
- Carbs: 50% of total calories

- Fat: Remaining calories after protein and carbs

I'll use myself as an example again for determining the calculations:

TDEE on high-carb days:

2,600 x .10= 260

2,600-260=2,340 total calories on high-carb days

Protein on high-carb days:

Your protein intake on high-carb days will simply be 1 gram of protein per pound of bodyweight:

1 gram per pound of bodyweight= 200 daily grams of protein

4 calories in 1 gram of protein x 200= 800 total calories from protein

Carbs on high-carb days:

To determine your carb intake on high-carb days, take your TDEE on high-carb days and multiply it by .5:

2,340 x .5= 1,170 total calories from carbs

You can then divide that number by 4 to get the gram equivalent:

1,170/4= 292.5 grams of carbs per day

Fat on high-carb days:

Your remaining calories will come from fat. Take your calculated TDEE, subtract your protein and carb calories from that number, and you'll be left with your calories from fat:

2,340 (TDEE)-800 (protein)-1,170 (carbs)=370 total calories from fat

You can then divide this number by 9 to get the gram equivalent:

370/9= 41.1 grams of fat per day

In summary, this would be my macros and calories on a high-carb day:

TDEE=2,340 calories
Protein= 200 grams (800 calories)
Carbs= 292.5 grams (1,170 calories)
Fat= 41.1 grams (370 calories)

You might be wondering why we're still eating 20% of our total calories from carbs on low-carb days. The reason why is because this is a low-carb day, not a no-carb day. Recall that carbs have many useful functions, and they're still making up a small percentage of the overall calories. It's high enough for you to keep your sanity (so you won't quit on the diet), but low enough for it to still be effective.

Then on your high-carb days, you're increasing your carb intake by *30%*—that's a big jump! It's definitely enough of a difference for your body to replenish leptin levels, which is exactly what we want. Going from 0% carbs to 50% would be too big of a leap, but a 30% increase hits the sweet spot.

You might also be wondering about protein. Why so much of it regardless of whether it's a high or low-carb day? You're consuming one gram of protein per pound of bodyweight for a couple of reasons:

#1: Protein has the highest thermic effect of food (TEF) of all 3 macronutrients.

The thermic effect of food is simply the amount of energy required to eat, digest, absorb and store food. Essentially, your body burns calories to digest the foods you eat!

Here's the approximate TEF for each macronutrient:

- Protein: 30-35%
- Carbs: 5-15%
- Fat: 3-4%

This means that if you consume 100 calories from protein, your body will burn roughly 30-35 calories to digest and process those original 100 calories. Conversely, if you consumed 100 calories from carbs, your body would only burn about 5-15 calories to digest and process the original 100 calories.

And since your calories are being restricted, it makes sense to consume high amounts of protein to maximize the TEF effect.

#2: Eating too little of protein when calories are restricted can lead to muscle loss

As you learned earlier, when you lower your calories for a prolonged period of time, your body will respond by slowing down your metabolism and holding onto body fat. Your body will still need energy to survive and function, so it'll get it by other means—i.e. your muscle mass. Fortunately, protein has a muscle-sparring effect (9), so if you consume enough of it, you'll be able to retain your lean muscle mass while dieting down. It won't do you any good to lose 20 pounds if 10 of those lost pounds were muscle.

Chapter 5: Carb Cycling and Building Muscle

Thus far, I've only talked about how you can use carb cycling as a way to lean down while retaining muscle mass. But what if your fitness goal is to build muscle? Can you still use carb cycling as a nutritional strategy to get the job done? The answer is yes, of course you can!

Carb cycling will make it easier for you to build muscle and at the same time minimize fat gain. It won't do you any good to bulk up and add 20 pounds to your frame if half of that weight is fat. You'll have to spend more time later cutting the fat you gained from the bulk!

What Changes When You Want to Build Muscle Instead of Burn Fat?

In terms of nutrition, the main thing that'll change when you want to build muscle is the amount of calories you eat. When your goal is to lose weight, you'll want to eat less calories than your total daily energy expenditure. When you want to build muscle, you'll want to consume more calories than your total daily energy expenditure. Calories are the building blocks your body will use to pack on lean muscle. Without enough calories, it won't be able to get the job done.

Think of it this way. Let's say you're a fisherman who wants to catch 100 fish in your net at a time. In order to do that, you'll need a net that's big enough to hold 100 fish in it. If your net can only hold 75 fish at a time then it won't be possible for you to reach your goal.

The same goes for calories and building muscle. For example, let's say your body needs 2,800 calories a day in order to build muscle. If you only eat 2,600 calories a day, then you're leaving muscle on the table because you're shorting your body of the necessary energy it needs to complete the task.

How Many Calories Do I Need to Eat to Start Building Muscle?

The key with calories and building muscle is to eat enough for your body to add mass, but not too much to where your body will store the excess calories as fat. You can't eat more and more and gain muscle in proportion to how much you're eating! Your body will use what it needs and then it'll store the rest as fat. That's why we want to eat right at that threshold where we'll add muscle but little to no fat.

To do that, we'll simply add 10% more calories to our total daily energy expenditure (TDEE).

Here's how to calculate it using myself as an example:

- 13 x bodyweight (200 pounds in my case)= TDEE of 2,600 calories

- 2,600 x .10= 260

- 260+2,600=2,860 total calories

This means that I'll need to eat 2,860 calories a day to build muscle with minimal fat gain.

Setting Up Your Carb Cycling Schedule

For fat loss, it's ideal to have a 3:1 low/high-carb ratio to maximize results. That is, for every 3 days you eat low-carbs, you'll have 1 day of high-carbs. To build muscle, we're going to change things up a bit. You're going to use a 3:2 low/high-carb ratio. For every 3 days you eat low-carbs, you'll have 2 days of eating high-carbs. The cool thing is that you don't have to do all of your low and high-carb days lined up in row, all though you can do that if you like.

Here are some different ways to set up your carb cycling schedule to build lean muscle mass:

Option #1:

- Monday: Low-carb day
- Tuesday: Low-carb day
- Wednesday: Low-carb day
- Thursday: High-carb day
- Friday: High-carb day
- Saturday: Low-carb day
- Sunday: Low-carb day
- Following Monday: Low-carb day, etc.

Option #2:

- Monday: High-carb day
- Tuesday: Low-carb day
- Wednesday: High-carb day
- Thursday: Low-carb day
- Friday: Low-carb day
- Saturday: High-carb day
- Sunday: Low-carb day
- Following Monday: High-carb day
- Following Tuesday: Low-carb day
- Following Wednesday: Low-carb day, etc.

Essentially with option #2, you'll have one high-carb day, one low-carb day, one high-carb day, 2 low-carb days, and then you'll repeat the cycle.

If you're having trouble determining what option you want to use for your cycle, consider your workout schedule (don't worry I'll cover a solid workout routine in chapter 6 if you need help with that). Ideally, you would want to have high-carb days on the same days that you workout. This is because on workout days your body will be burning more calories, and it'll need the extra carbs to help fuel the workout and start the recovery process.

On your rest days, you'll be burning less overall calories, and thus the carbs won't be needed as much. Of course, you won't always be able to time it to where you workout on the same day as a high-carb day, but you'll want to align it up as much as you can.

Macro Percentages for High and Low-Carb Days

These calculations won't be too much different from the ones we used when the goal was weight loss. The two main differences are that you'll be consuming a higher percentage of your calories from carbs and that you'll be eating more total calories.

Macro Percentages for Low-Carb Days to Build Muscle

Consume the following macros and calories during your low-carb days to build muscle:

- Total calories: Consume 10% more calories than your total daily energy expenditure (TDEE)
- Protein: 1 gram per pound of bodyweight
- Carbs: 25% of total calories

- Fat: Remaining calories after protein and carbs

I'll use myself as an example for determining the calculations:

TDEE on low-carb days:

2,600 x .10= 260

2,600+260=2,860 total daily calories on low-carb days

Protein on low-carb days:

Your protein intake on low-carb days will simply be 1 gram of protein per pound of bodyweight:

1 gram per pound of bodyweight= 200 daily grams of protein

4 calories in 1 gram of protein x 200= 800 total calories from protein

Carbs on low-carb days:

To determine your carb intake on low-carb days, take your TDEE on low-carb days and multiply it by .25:

2,860 x .25= 715 total calories from carbs

You can then divide that number by 4 to get the gram equivalent:

715/4= 178.75 grams of carbs per day

Fat on low-carb days:

Your remaining calories will come from fat. Take your calculated TDEE, subtract your protein and carb calories from that number, and you'll be left with your calories from fat:

2,860 (TDEE)-800 (protein)-715 (carbs)=1,345 total calories from fat

You can then divide this number by 9 to get the gram equivalent:

1,345/9= 149.4 grams of fat per day

In summary, this would be my macros and calories on a low-carb day to build muscle:

TDEE=2,860 calories
Protein= 200 grams (800 calories)
Carbs= 178.75 grams (715 calories)
Fat= 149.4 grams (1,345 calories)

Macro Percentages for High-Carb Days to Build Muscle

Consume the following macros and calories on your high-carb days to build muscle:

- Total calories: Consume 10% more calories than your total daily energy expenditure (TDEE). And yes, this means your TDEE will be the same on low and high-carb days!
- Protein: 1 gram per pound of bodyweight
- Carbs: 50% of total calories
- Fat: Remaining calories after protein and carbs

I'll use myself as an example again for determining the calculations:

TDEE on high-carb days:

2,600 x .10= 260

2,600+260=2,860 total calories on high-carb days

Protein on high-carb days:

Your protein intake on high-carb days will simply be 1 gram of protein per pound of bodyweight:

1 gram per pound of bodyweight= 200 daily grams of protein

4 calories in 1 gram of protein x 200= 800 total calories from protein

Carbs on high-carb days:

To determine your carb intake on high-carb days, take your TDEE on high-carb days and multiply it by .5:

2,860 x .50= 1,430 total calories from carbs

You can then divide that number by 4 to get the gram equivalent:

1,430/4= 357.5 grams of carbs per day

Fat on high-carb days:

Your remaining calories will come from fat. Take your calculated TDEE, subtract your protein and carb calories from that number, and you'll be left with your calories from fat:

2,860 (TDEE)-800 (protein)-1,430 (carbs)=630 total calories from fat

You can then divide this number by 9 to get the gram equivalent:

630/9= 70 grams of fat per day

In summary, this would be my macros and calories on a high-carb day:

TDEE=2,860 calories
Protein= 200 grams (800 calories)
Carbs= 357.5 grams (1,430 calories)
Fat= 70 grams (630 calories)

Chapter 6: Muscle Building Workout With Carb Cycling

Exercise is very important not only for your health but also for determining how your physique will look. If you want to build your best body possible, you must incorporate resistance training into your overall fitness plan. If you only use diet to lean down, something won't look quite right when you reach your goal bodyweight. Sure you'll have a low body fat percentage, but you'll end up looking flat, skinny and weak.

Resistance training is what stimulates your muscles to grow. However, your muscles don't actually grow when you're working out. During the workout, you're breaking down your muscle cells and telling your body to start the process of rebuilding them. It's during the recovery process, when you're getting plenty of rest and eating the right foods that your damaged muscles will start to grow back bigger and stronger.

Working out is what will get you a lean and defined look. Whether you're male or female, you don't have to overdue it and take on the look of an overly bulky bodybuilder. Additionally, weight training will also help prevent muscle loss (10). It basically comes down to the "use it or lose it" principle. If you restrict your calories and you aren't weight training, your body won't have any use for extra muscle, and it's more likely to use it for energy. Conversely, if you regularly lift weights, your body will keep that additional muscle mass because it knows that it'll need it sooner or later.

Workout to Build Muscle Mass Fast

The following training routine will consist of two different workouts—workout A and workout B. You'll alternate between workout A and workout B every time you go to the gym. You can workout 3 or 4 days per week; either way will get you results, so pick what works best for your schedule.

Here's how to set up your gym schedule if you want to workout three days per week:

Monday: Workout A
Tuesday: Rest Day
Wednesday: Workout B
Thursday: Rest Day
Friday: Workout A
Saturday: Rest Day
Sunday: Rest Day
Following Monday: Workout B

Or:

Monday: Rest Day
Tuesday: Workout A
Wednesday: Rest Day
Thursday: Workout B
Friday: Rest Day
Saturday: Workout A
Sunday: Rest Day
Following Tuesday: Workout B

And here's how to set up your gym schedule if you want to workout 4 days per week:

Monday: Workout A
Tuesday: Workout B

Wednesday: Rest Day
Thursday: Workout A
Friday: Workout B
Saturday: Rest Day
Sunday: Rest Day

Or:

Monday: Workout A
Tuesday: Workout B
Wednesday: Rest Day
Thursday: Workout A
Friday: Rest Day
Saturday: Workout B
Sunday: Rest Day

The second option will give your central nervous system an extra day of rest in-between your third and fourth workouts, which you may find beneficial. In the end though, pick whatever option works best for you and is the easiest for you to stick with.

Here are the actual workouts:

Workout A: Chest, Shoulders, and Triceps

- Incline Barbell or Dumbbell Bench Press: 3 sets of 6 reps 3 min rest btw (between) sets
- Standing Barbell Military Press: 3 sets of 6 reps 3 min rest btw sets
- Overhead Dumbbell Triceps Extension: 3 sets of 8 reps 90 sec rest btw sets
- Seated Dumbbell Lateral Raises: 3 sets of 10-12 reps 60 sec rest btw sets
- Face Pulls: 3 sets of 10-12 reps 60 sec rest btw sets
- Tricep Rope Pushdown: 3 sets of 12 reps 60 sec rest btw sets

Workout B: Back, Biceps, and Legs

- Weighted Pull-Ups (replace with lat pulldowns if you're unable to do pull-ups): 3 sets of 6 reps 3 min rest btw sets
- Barbell Back Squats: 3 sets of 8 reps 2 min rest btw sets
- Standing Dumbbell Curls: 3 sets of 8 reps 90 sec rest btw sets
- Bent Over Row: 3 sets of 8 reps 2 min rest btw sets
- Cross Body Hammer Curls: 3 sets of 10-12 reps 60 sec rest btw sets

Side Note: A set is a group of consecutive repetitions. A repetition is one complete motion of an exercise. And the rest period is how long of a break you'll take until you start the next set. For example, let's say you're completing 3 sets of 8 reps and resting 2 minutes in between sets for the barbell back squat exercise.

You'll squat down and stand back up, completing the motion of the exercise and one rep. You'll repeat that motion 7 more times for a total of 8 repetitions. That will complete the set and you will begin your rest period. Once your 2-minute rest period is up, you'll start the next set and perform another 8 repetitions.

That will complete set number 2, and you'll rest another 2 minutes. Once that time period is up, you'll complete the final set of 8 repetitions, and then you'll move onto the next exercise.

One of the reasons why I love this workout so much is because of the frequency. You'll be training each muscle group twice per week. This is important because muscle protein synthesis is increased in a muscle group for up to 48 hours after you train it (11). Muscle protein synthesis is the rate at which protein is being shuttled into and out of a particular muscle.

With a typical bro split, you'd be working out five days a week, and you'd only be training one muscle group per workout. The workout is typically set up like this:

Monday: Chest
Tuesday: Back
Wednesday: Legs
Thursday: Shoulders
Friday: Arms
Saturday: Rest Day
Sunday: Rest Day

The problem with this workout split is that you're only working out each muscle group one time per week! When you workout your chest on Monday, muscle protein synthesis will be increased in that area for 48 hours. Instead of training your chest again once that 48-hour period is up, you'll be waiting around for another four days before you workout chest again!

Who do you think would add more muscle to his chest over the course of a year?

Person A who works out his chest once a week for a total of 52 times a year.

Or:

Person B who works out his chest twice per week for a total of 104 times per year.

The answer is obvious. The reason why bro splits are so popular is because so many bodybuilders use them. However, there many be more to that than meets the eye and sometimes drugs could be a part of the equation.

Certain substances help them recover from their workouts faster than natural lifters like you and I. So while a bro split may be a good idea for a substance abusing bodybuilder, it has little use for us. Stick with the workout plan and get stronger with the given exercises. That's the best way to make gains quickly!

Chapter 7: What About Cardio?

Cardio is a very hot topic in the fitness community today. You hear about professional bodybuilders using it to lean down for competitions, but then you hear someone else bashing it for being too slow and boring.

So who's right in all of this? Hopefully, I can set you on the right path and give you a true understanding of what cardio is all about.

Is Cardio Even Necessary to Lose Weight?

The answer to the above question is definitely not! I can completely understand why many people think that they must do hours upon hours of cardio if they want to shred a few pounds. You hear all of the time about how fitness models and bodybuilders use cardio as a way to get absolutely shredded, so it's easy to believe it's required. However, cardio is not required at all to lose weight and get down to a low level of body fat.

What is required to lose weight and shred fat is eating less calories than your total daily energy expenditure as I mentioned earlier. It doesn't matter if you use exercise (i.e. cardio in this case) and/or diet to achieve that, both will get the job done. With that being said, it's much easier to control your total number of calories through your diet as opposed to exercising more. Think about it for a second.

What's easier- eating a slice of pizza and then doing 30 minutes of cardio to burn it off or not eating the slice of pizza in the first place? It's obvious; you shouldn't eat the pizza in the first place. Sure, you could try to burn off the extra calories every now and then, but it won't last for long. You're fighting an uphill battle because 30 minutes of your time isn't worth whatever it is that you want to eat so badly.

That's why you hear people say that you can't out exercise a bad diet. It's true, so focus more on your diet and the number of calories that you're eating instead of doing more cardio. Also, don't fret if you think this means that you'll have to give up your favorite foods to lose weight because it doesn't. You'll still get to enjoy your favorite foods *without* having to worry about weight gain or doing some extra cardio to make up for it.

How You Should Think About Cardio

From now on, I want you to think about cardio as a tool that can help you burn some extra calories instead of thinking of cardio as a requirement to do with carb cycling to lose weight. Cardio is one way to help get you below your total daily energy expenditure (TDEE), and you can use it when you feel that it's needed to get the job done.

As a single tool usually won't be enough to get the job done, cardio alone usually won't be enough to get you burning more calories than your TDEE. The main focus still needs to be on the carb cycling nutrition plan I outlined earlier. With this type of mindset, you'll only have to do cardio when you feel that it's necessary. It's important to note that moderate to high intensity cardio *isn't required* at all for carb cycling to work.

I believe that honing in on nutrition is the right way to go when trying to lose weight. This is because diet is the easiest and fastest way to control the total number of calories you're eating. However, once you have your diet in check, if you feel like adding in some extra exercise, then by all means do so. Cardio can be a good way to speed up the fat loss process or at the very least give you some more leeway in your diet.

The Best Cardio Workout

With so many cardio workouts in existence today, which one is the best? Is it a slow steady state cardio? How about sprinting? Or maybe any type of cardio done on an empty stomach is the best?

The kind of cardio that you do doesn't matter much. This is because if the cardio workout doesn't put your total caloric intake below your TDEE (I know I keep bringing this up so it must be important, right?), then you won't be losing any weight.

So I would first and foremost recommend doing any type of cardio you enjoy whether that's walking, sprinting, jogging, swimming, kickboxing, etc. However, I will say the cardio workout I'll be providing you with here is the best way to go. It's a combination of high intensity interval training (HIIT) and slow steady state cardio. Research has shown higher intensity cardio results in more fat loss over time than lower intensity cardio (12) (13).

HIIT really is efficient—you're burning more calories in less time. HIIT's even cooler though when combined with slow steady state cardio. The reason why is because the HIIT will release free fatty acids into the bloodstream, and then the slow steady state cardio will burn off those free fatty acids.

Most people will do HIIT but won't follow it up with slow steady state cardio. This is a shame because all of those free fatty acids released into the bloodstream will get reabsorbed.

Here's how to do a combo cardio workout:

Note: This cardio workout can be done on any type of cardio machine (treadmill, elliptical, etc.), outside, on a track or wherever else you want. No matter where you are, the workout will be the same.

Combo Cardio Workout

#1: 10-15 minutes of HIIT on treadmill (or cardio machine of choice)

    -Sprint for 30 seconds

    -Walk for 1 minute (alternate between sprinting and walking for the full 10-15 min)

#2: Immediately followed by: 10-15 minutes of steady state cardio

    -Walk on treadmill at 3.5 mph

Now the cool thing about HIIT is that you can adjust it to your current fitness level. For example if you can't sprint for 30 seconds, do a fast jog for 20 seconds (7.5 mph on a treadmill as an example) and then walk for 1 minute and 10 seconds.

You could even do 45 seconds of sprinting and 45 seconds of walking if you're in better shape. You can customize it to your needs, but you have the do the HIIT first followed by the slow steady state cardio.

I recommend that you do this 20-30 minute workout 2 times per week. I wouldn't advise that you do it anymore than 2 times per week because that's too much and it's not necessary beyond that point.

Final Cardio Considerations

Here's the deal:

You might not feel like doing HIIT sometimes. What do you do then? Luckily, you don't have to skip cardio altogether—

there's an easier way and it's called walking. I recommend walking as much as you possibly can.

Walking is great because it can help to reduce stress (14) and speed up recovery from a hard workout. Walking also helps with lymphatic system recovery, and there's research showing how walking more (or moving more in general for that matter) can reduce your risk for developing heart disease (15).

Best of all, walking is an easy way to burn more calories. I used to think that walking was only for people who weren't in that good of shape, but boy was I wrong about that! Walking should be done by everyone, fit or unfit. The simple fact is that walking provides benefits that the higher intensity cardio can't.

I recommend going for walks around town or at the local park. Go outside and get some fresh air. Walking for 30 minutes 3 days a week would be enough to start providing you with some amazing benefits. You can still do the combination cardio workout twice per week in addition to the walking if you want to.

Chapter 8: 30 Low-Carb Recipes

Tilapia Parmesan

Ingredients:

- 2- 6 oz. tilapia fillets
- 2 tbsp. mayonnaise
- 2 tbsp. plain yogurt
- 1/4 cup parmesan cheese
- 3 sprigs fresh dill
- 1 tsp. garlic powder
- Black pepper to taste

Directions:

1. Put mayonnaise, yogurt and parmesan cheese in a small bowl and mix with a spoon.
2. Cover a cookie sheet with aluminum and spray with cooking spray.
3. Put oven to broil on high.
4. Put tilapia fillets roughly 2 inches apart on cookie sheet.
5. Divide cheese mixture evenly on each fillet.
6. Rub dill with fingers to separate roughly 1.5 sprigs worth of leaves over each fillet.
7. Sprinkle each fillet with half of garlic powder and season with salt and pepper.
8. Place cookie sheet into broiler.
9. Cook for 7-10 minutes, let cool and enjoy!

Number of servings: 2

Macros (per serving):

Calories: 275.2
Protein: 48.5 g
Carbs: 1.4 g
Fat: 8.5 g

*Recipe courtesy of LEXIBELLE715

Lime Chicken

Ingredients:

- 4 skinless and boneless chicken breasts
- 3 garlic cloves
- 1 cup salsa
- 1 1/2 worth lime juice
- 1/4 cup reduced fat ranch dressing
- 1 cup reduced fat cheddar cheese

Directions:

1. Spray skillet with cooking heat and place stove on medium heat.
2. Chop chicken breasts in half.
3. Sauté chicken for 3 minutes per side.
4. Add in garlic.
5. In a separate bowl, mix salsa, lime juice and ranch dressing.
6. Spread mixture onto the chicken.
7. Cook for another 5 minutes.
8. Add in the cheese and cook for another 5 minutes until chicken is no longer pink.

Number of servings: 8

Macros (per serving):

Calories: 208.9
Protein: 31.4 g
Carbs: 6.7 g
Fata: 6.2 g

*Recipe courtesy of VJB2601

Tuna Salad

Ingredients:

- 1 can albacore tuna
- 2/3 cup non-fat cottage cheese
- 4 tbsp. plain low-fat yogurt
- 1/4 small red onion, finely chopped
- 1 stalk celery, finely chopped
- 1 tsp. Dijon mustard
- Squirt of lemon juice
- A pinch of dill

Directions:

1. Mix all of the ingredients in a bowl and enjoy!

Number of servings: 2

Macros (per serving):

Calories: 190.3
Protein: 32.5 g
Carbs: 11.7 g
Fat: 2.2 g

*Recipe courtesy of GORGEOUS26

Parmesan Shrimp

Ingredients:

- 14 medium shrimp, peeled and deveined
- 1 tbsp. olive oil
- 1/2 clove garlic, minced
- 2 dashes of salt
- 1/4 tsp. Creole seasoning
- 2 dashes of ground pepper
- 1/8 cup Panko breadcrumbs
- 1 tbsp. shredded parmesan cheese

Directions:

1. Place shrimp, garlic, olive oil, salt, pepper and Creole seasoning into Ziploc bag.
2. Flip bag in multiple directions until shrimp is well coated.
3. Place in fridge for 1.5 hours.
4. Preheat oven to 475 degrees F.
5. Add bread crumbs and Parmesan to bag and turn until coated.
6. Spray a baking pan with butter and arrange shrimp on pan to where they don't touch.
7. Broil for roughly 10 minutes or until thoroughly cooked.
8. Add in the squeezed lemon and enjoy!

Number of servings: 2

Macros (per serving):

Calories: 137.6
Protein: 10.2 g
Carbs: 4.7 g
Fat: 8.6 g
*Recipe courtesy of PRAIRIEHARPY

Crustless Quiche

Ingredients:

- 1 cup non-fat cottage cheese
- 2 cups liquid egg whites
- 1/2 cup cooled broccoli
- 1/2 cup ham
- 1/2 cup low-fat Colby cheese
- Salt and pepper to taste

Directions:

1. Preheat oven to 375 degrees F.
2. Mix all of the ingredients into a large bowl.
3. Spray a pie dish with cooking spray.
4. Put mixture into pie dish.
5. Put dish into oven, bake for 45 minutes and enjoy!

Number of servings: 6

Macros (per serving):

Calories: 106.8
Protein: 18.7 g
Carbs: 4.5 g
Fat: 1.4 g

*Recipe courtesy of CHESSMANS2000

Chicken Burgers

Ingredients:

- 1 lb. ground chicken
- 6 oz. crumbled feta
- 1 tbsp. ground oregano
- 1/4 tsp. salt
- 1/4 tsp. garlic powder

Directions:

1. Preheat broiler or grill.
2. Mix all of the ingredients together and form into 4 separate patties.
3. Grill or broil patties until internal temperature of burgers reaches 165 degrees F (approximately 8 minutes per side).
4. Serve and enjoy!

Number of servings: 4

Macros (per serving):

Calories: 285.6
Protein: 26.8 g
Carbs: 3.3 g
Fat: 19.8 g

*Recipe courtesy of PRAIRIEHARPY

Salmon Cakes

Ingredients:

- 1 can wild Alaskan Pink Salmon
- 1 cup raw onion
- 1 tsp. black pepper
- 1 tsp. garlic powder
- 1 large egg
- salt to taste

Directions:

1. Mix all of the ingredients together.
2. For mixture into 4 separate patties.
3. Fry patties similar to the way you would a burger until thoroughly cooked.

Number of servings: 4

Macros (per serving):

Calories: 195.0
Protein: 23.2 g
Carbs: 4.5 g
Fat: 10.1 g

*Recipe courtesy of MYTHINKER

Teriyaki Meatballs

Ingredients:

- 1 lb. lean ground beef
- 1/2 cup chopped green onions
- 1/3 cup teriyaki sauce
- 3 tsp. chopped ginger root

Directions:

1. Preheat oven to 350 degrees F.
2. Mix all of the ingredients together in a separate bowl.
3. Form 8- 2 oz. balls with the mixture.
4. Place the balls into a dish and bake for 25-30 minutes.

Number of servings: 8

Macros (per serving):

Calories: 101.1
Protein: 13.1 g
Carbs: 3.8 g
Fat: 3.5 g

*Recipe courtesy of PRAIRIEHARPY

Chicken Alfredo Bake

Ingredients:

- 3 boneless skinless chicken breasts
- 1 tbsp. cooking oil
- Montreal seasoning
- 1 cup cubed yellow squash
- 1 medium diced sweet onion
- 1 cup cauliflower
- salt and pepper to taste
- 1 jar Alfredo sauce
- 1/4 cup grated parmesan cheese
- 1/8 cup bread crumbs

Directions:

1. Preheat oven to 350 degrees F.
2. Spray 13x9 pan with cooking spray.
3. Sprinkle Montreal seasoning over chicken breasts and cook in skillet until there's no pink.
4. Put cauliflower in dish, add 2 tbsp. water, cover with plastic wrap and cook in microwave for 4 minutes.
5. Sauté cooking oil and onions until clear. Add in squash and sauté until soft.
6. Cut chicken into cubes and add to casserole dish with vegetable. Pour Alfredo sauce over the top of dish.
7. Top with cheese and bread crumbs and bake for 20 minutes, and then boil for 10 until top of dish is brown.

Number of servings: 8

Macros (per serving):

Calories: 240.1
Protein: 26.9 g
Carbs: 6.9 g

Fat: 12.0 g

*Recipe courtesy of PRAIRIEHARPY

Lettuce Wraps

Ingredients:

- 3.5 oz. lean ground beef
- 1 tbsp. finely minced onion
- 1 clove crushed minced garlic
- Dash garlic powder
- Dash dried oregano
- Chopped cilantro to taste
- Cayenne pepper to taste
- Salt and pepper to taste
- Lettuce leaves

Directions:

1. Brown ground beef until thoroughly cooked.
2. Add onion, garlic, spices, and a little water and simmer for 7-10 minutes.
3. Add salt to taste.
4. Add mixture onto lettuce, wrap it up, and enjoy!

Number of servings: 1

Macros (per serving):

Calories: 143.5
Protein: 21.7 g
Carbs: 4.2 g
Fat: 1.4 g

*Recipe courtesy of LIZZY63

Scrambled Eggs

Ingredients:

- 1/4 cup green bell pepper, finely chopped
- 1 tbsp. onion, finely chopped
- 2 large eggs
- 1/4 cup low-fat cottage cheese
- 2 tbsp. low-fat cheddar cheese
- 2 tbsp. salsa

Directions:

1. Beat eggs and cottage cheese together.
2. Spray nonstick skillet with cooking spray.
3. Cook peppers and onions on medium heat until tender, roughly 2 minutes.
4. Add egg mixture and cheddar cheese.
5. Reduce heat to medium. Cook until set, stirring as needed.
6. Put the salsa on top and enjoy!

Number of servings: 1

Macros (per serving):

Calories: 274.8
Protein: 24.3 g
Carbs: 7.9 g
Fat: 14.5 g

*Recipe courtesy of SOOKIE

Pork Chops for Crockpot

Ingredients:

- 10 pork chops
- 1 can low fat chicken cream soup
- 1/2 cup ketchup

Directions:

1. Put the pork chops into the crockpot.
2. Add in the soup and ketchup.
3. Cover the crockpot and cook on low for 8-9 hours.
4. Serve and enjoy!

Number of servings: 10

Macros (per serving):

Calories: 239.7
Protein: 21.8 g
Carbs: 8.2 g
Fat: 12.1 g

*Recipe courtesy of LASTX70

Country Style Crockpot Pork Ribs

Ingredients:

- 1/4 tsp. ground allspice
- 1/4 tsp. ground cinnamon
- 2 pounds country-style pork ribs
- 1/4 cup diced onion
- 1/2 tsp. garlic powder
- 1 tbsp. sugar-free maple-flavored syrup
- 1 dash black pepper
- 1/4 tsp. ground ginger
- 1 tbsp. low-sodium soy sauce

Directions:

1. Mix all of the ingredients into a bowl minus the ribs.
2. Pour mixture over ribs.
3. Put ribs in crockpot and cook for 8-9 hours on low.
4. Cover with foil and bake for 60-90 minutes if baking in oven.

Number of servings: 4

Macros (per serving):

Calories: 188.4
Protein: 22.3 g
Carbs: 2.3 g
Fat: 9.4 g

*Recipe courtesy of LANDMOM

Cottage Cheese Breakfast

Ingredients:

- 1 cup 1% cottage cheese
- 1 tsp. ground cinnamon
- 1 packet Splenda
- 1/4 cup chopped almonds

Directions:

1. Put the cottage cheese, cinnamon, and Splenda in a bowl and mix well.
2. Sprinkle the chopped almonds on top and enjoy!

Number of servings: 1

Macros (per serving):

Calories: 249.8
Protein: 30.8 g
Carbs: 14.9 g
Fat: 8.6 g

*Recipe courtesy of NURSEHOPE

Tuna Burgers

Ingredients:

- 2 cups tuna
- 1/3 cup tomato sauce
- 1/4 cup finely chopped dill pickle onions
- 2 egg whites
- 1/4 cup wholegrain flour
- 1/4 tsp. black pepper
- 1/2 tsp. garlic powder
- 1/2 tsp. onion powder

Directions:

1. Put all of the ingredients in a bowl and thoroughly mix together.
2. Form mixture into 4 separate patties.
3. Spray skillet with cooking spray and cook on medium-high heat until thoroughly cooked on each side.
4. Serve and enjoy!

Number of servings: 4

Macros (per serving):

Calories: 140.5
Protein: 23.7 g
Carbs: 8.5 g
Fat: 1.3 g

*Recipe courtesy of FLOWERDALEJEWEL

Cheddar Bread

Ingredients:

- 1 large egg
- 2 tsp. flax seed meal
- 1/2 tbsp. baking powder
- 1 packet Splenda
- 1/4 cup shredded cheddar cheese
- 1 tsp. melted butter

Directions:

1. Melt butter in flat bowl or 15 oz. oval ramekin.
2. Add in the egg, flax meal, baking powder, Splenda, cheddar cheese and mix well.
3. Put in the microwave for 1 minute.
4. Flip over and cook for another 10 seconds until cooked throughout.
5. Cut in half, serve with favorite sandwich fillings and enjoy!

Number of servings: 1

Macros (per serving):

Calories: 289.2
Protein: 16.4 g
Carbs: 5.4 g
Fat: 22.5 g

*Recipe courtesy of XANADUREALM

Scampi Shrimp

Ingredients:

- 1 tbsp. canola oil
- 3/4 lb. uncooked peeled and deveined shrimp
- 1 med diced green onion
- 1/4 tsp. garlic powder
- 1/2 tsp. basil
- 3/4 tsp. parsley
- 1 tbsp. lemon juice
- 3 tbsp. parmesan cheese

Directions:

1. Heat oil over medium heat in 10" skillet.
2. Add shrimp and remaining ingredients to skillet.
3. Cook for 5-7 minutes.
4. Remove skillet from heat and sprinkle with Parmesan cheese.
5. Serve and enjoy!

Number of servings: 4

Macros (per serving):

Calories: 143.5
Protein: 19.0 g
Carbs: 2.1 g
Fat: 6.1 g

*Recipe courtesy of JOELSANGEL

No-Carb Cajun Tilapia

Ingredients:

- 4 oz. tilapia filet
- 1 tsp. extra virgin olive oil
- 1/2 tbsp. unsalted butter
- Favorite Cajun spice of your choosing to taste

Directions:

1. Melt butter and olive oil in a skillet.
2. Cover fish with Cajun spice.
3. Cook fish fillet in butter and oil for 3-5 minutes per side until thoroughly cooked.
4. Serve and enjoy!

Number of servings: 1

Macros (per serving):

Calories: 143.9
Protein: 21.0 g
Carbs: 0.0 g
Fat: 6.3 g

*Recipe courtesy of THEBERT99

Regular Chicken Salad

Ingredients:

- 1 1/2 cups cooked and chopped chicken
- 1 1/2 cups chopped celery
- 3 tbsp. light mayonnaise
- 1 tsp. mustard
- Salt and pepper to taste

Directions:

1. Put all of the ingredients together in a bowl and thoroughly mix together.

Number of servings: 1

Macros (per serving):

Calories: 173.8
Protein: 24.2 g
Carbs: 3.5 g
Fat: 6.3 g

*Recipe courtesy of JTDALZELL

Chocolate Cheesecake

Ingredients:

For Sauce:
- 2 tbsp. butter
- 4 tbsp. cocoa
- 3 tbsp. Splenda

For Cake:
- 16 oz. cream cheese
- 1 pkg. of sugar free instant chocolate pudding mix
- 1/2 cup of heavy cream
- 1/2 cup of Splenda
- 1 tsp. vanilla extract
- 2 eggs

Directions:

For Sauce:

1. Melt together butter, cocoa and Splenda (3 tbsp. worth) on stovetop or in microwave.

For Cake:

1. Preheat oven to 350 degrees F.
2. Mix together cream cheese, Splenda, vanilla and eggs.
3. Mix heavy cream and pudding together in separate bowl from other mixture.
4. Combine both mixtures toughly in blender.
5. Spray a pie plate with cooking spray.
6. Put cheesecake mixture in pan and place in oven for around 40 minutes.
7. Remove and drizzle sauce on top. Refrigerate, serve cold and enjoy!

Number of servings: 12

Macros (per serving):

Calories: 207.7
Protein: 4.8 g
Carbs: 5.4 g
Fat: 20.0 g

*Recipe courtesy of JNORMAN1969

Cauliflower Faux Mashed Potatoes

Ingredients:

- 1 head raw cauliflower (5-6 in. in diameter)
- 1/4 cup sour cream
- 2 tbsp. salted butter

Directions:

1. Steam cauliflower until soft.
2. Put cooked cauliflower in a pot and heat to get rid of the excess moisture.
3. Puree cauliflower in food processor.
4. Add butter and sour cream and enjoy!

Number of servings: 4

Macros (per serving):

Calories: 117.6
Protein: 3.4 g
Carbs: 8.1 g
Fat: 9.1 g

*Recipe courtesy of ARTEMISINKED

Chicken Noodle Soup

Ingredients:

- 1 package fettuccini noodles
- 1 cup chopped onion
- 1 cup chopped cabbage
- 1 cup spinach
- 1 cup chopped carrots
- 1 clove garlic
- 1 tsp. ginger
- 1 tsp. red pepper flakes
- 8 oz. chicken
- 4 cups broth
- 1 tbsp. soy sauce

Directions:

1. Rinse fettuccini noodles under warm water for 30 seconds, drain, and let air dry while preparing other ingredients.
2. Boil the 4 cups of broth.
3. Add all of the ingredients to the broth (noodles included) and cook for 6-7 minutes until vegetables become tender.

Number of servings: 4

Macros (per serving):

Calories: 174.5
Protein: 18.8 g
Carbs: 11.8 g
Fat: 6.1 g

*Recipe courtesy of CLYNNTHOMAS

Beef and Turkey Meatloaf

Ingredients:

- 3 1/2 lbs. ground turkey
- 3 1/2 lbs. ground beef
- 1 cup chopped onion
- 1 cup shredded carrots
- 1 sleeve saltine crackers
- 1/2 cup non-fat milk
- 4 large eggs
- 1 tbsp. salt
- 1 tbsp. pepper
- 2 tbsp. Worcestershire sauce
- 6 chopped cloves of garlic

Directions:

1. Preheat oven to 350 degrees F.
2. In a large bowl, crumble up the crackers and soak them in the milk for 15 minutes.
3. Chop the vegetables and add remaining ingredients to the cracker bowl.
4. Mix all of the ingredients in the bowl together until combined.
5. Form the combined mixture into a rectangle load in a 13x9 baking dish.
6. Bake for 80-90 minutes or until internal temp. reaches 160 degrees.
7. Cool for 10 minutes, serve, and enjoy!

Number of servings: 12

Macros (per serving):

Calories: 467.1
Protein: 21.7 g
Carbs: 8.5 g

Fat: 31.7 g

*Recipe courtesy of CLYNNTHOMAS

Chicken Enchiladas

Ingredients:

- 2 skinless chicken breasts
- 1 can cream chicken soup
- 1 can cream mushroom soup
- 1/4 cup diced green chilies
- 1 cup salsa verde
- 1/4 cup chopped tomatoes
- 8 whole-wheat tortillas
- 2 cups Colby jack cheese

Directions:

1. Preheat oven to 350 degrees F.
2. Boil the chicken breast and shred when cooled.
3. Mix cream chicken and cream mushroom soups, cheese, chilies, salsa verde and tomatoes together in large bowl.
4. Remove half of the mixture from the bowl and set aside for later use.
5. Add shredded chicken remaining mixture in bowl.
6. Lay a tortilla flat and fill with about 3 tsp. of the chicken, then repeat this process for the remaining tortillas.
7. Pour the rest of the mixture you set aside earlier over the top of the enchiladas and bake for 45 minutes.
8. Cool for 15 minutes and enjoy!

Number of servings: 8

Macros (per serving):

Calories: 155.4
Protein: 13.9 g

Carbs: 4.2 g
Fat: 7.3 g

*Recipe courtesy of KFOX05

Protein Shake

Ingredients:

- 1 scoop (roughly 33 grams) vanilla cream whey protein powder
- 8 oz. unsweetened almond breeze vanilla almond milk
- 6 ice cubes
- 1 tsp. of vanilla extract

Directions:

1. Put all of the ingredients together in a blender and blend until smooth.

Number of servings: 1

Macros (per serving):

Calories: 170.0
Protein: 24.0 g
Carbs: 8.0 g
Fat: 4.5 g

*Recipe courtesy of LISAM67

Veggie Bacon Cheese Omlet

Ingredients:

- 1/4 cup liquid egg whites
- 1/4 cup raw onions
- 1/4 cup chopped green peppers
- 1/4 cup chopped tomatoes
- 1/4 cup reduced fat feta cheese
- 1/4 serving pre-cooked bacon

Directions:

1. Spray skillet with cooking spray and place on medium heat.
2. Add in peppers and onions and sauté for a bit until crisp.
3. Tear apart the bacon and add to skillet.
4. Add in the egg mixture and mix together with other ingredients.
5. Put the tomatoes and feta cheese on top and continue stirring until done.

Number of servings: 1

Macros (per serving):

Calories: 170.3
Protein: 20.3 g
Carbs: 9.6 g
Fat: 4.9 g

*Recipe courtesy of NATNEAGLE

Pumpkin Spice Frappuccino

Ingredients:

- 3/4 tsp. pumpkin spice
- 1-2 tsp. instant coffee
- 3 tbsp. canned pumpkin
- 1 tsp. stevia
- 2 tsp. sugar twin
- 3 tbsp. French vanilla coffee creamer
- 1 cup unsweetened coconut milk
- 6 ice cubes

Directions:

1. Put all of the ingredients in a blender and blend until mixture is smooth.

Number of servings: 2

Macros (per serving):

Calories: 66.3
Protein: 0.6 g
Carbs: 3.3 g
Fat: 4.7 g

*Recipe courtesy of MISTYRIOS

Taco Salad

Ingredients:

- 1 lb. extra lean ground beef
- 1 pkg. old El Paso taco seasoning
- 3/4 cup water
- 2 tbsp. olive oil
- 4 cups shredded romaine lettuce
- 1/2 cup chopped tomatoes
- 8 tbsp. fat free sour cream
- 1 cup shredded cheddar cheese

Directions:

1. Chop lettuce and set aside with tomatoes, cheese and sour cream.
2. Brown the beef with olive oil in skillet until thoroughly cooked.
3. Add in the taco seasoning and water to the skillet.
4. Simmer until water is reduced and remove from heat when done.
5. In 4 bowls, put one cup of lettuce in each bowl.
6. Add ¼ cup chopped tomatoes, beef, and cheese to each bowl.
7. Then add two tbsp. of sour cream to each bowl, serve and enjoy!

Number of servings: 4

Macros (per serving):

Calories: 489.0
Protein: 31.0 g
Carbs: 9.6 g
Fat: 36.1 g

*Recipe courtesy of TOASTERGIRL

Snicker doodle Cookies

Ingredients:

- 1/2 cup butter
- 1 1/2 cup almond flour
- 1 cup Splenda
- 1 egg
- 1/2 tsp. vanilla
- 1/4 tsp. baking soda
- 1/4 tsp. cream of tartar
- 2 tbs. Splenda
- 1 tsp. cinnamon

Directions:

1. Mix together all of the ingredients minus the cinnamon and Splenda.
2. Cover the bowl and refrigerate for 1 hour.
3. In a separate bowl, mix together the cinnamon and Splenda.
4. Roll dough in small balls throughout Splenda and cinnamon mixture.
5. Place dough balls on mixture and bake in oven at 350 degrees F for 15 minutes.
6. Remove and cool for 10 minutes and enjoy!

Number of servings: 20

Macros (per serving):

Calories: 99.1
Protein: 2.5 g
Carbs: 4.4 g
Fat: 9.4 g

*Recipe courtesy of SHELLSLYN

Chile Casserole

Ingredients:

- 2- 7 oz. cans of green chilies
- 8 oz. shredded pepper-jack cheese
- 3 eggs
- 3/4 cup heavy cream
- 1/2 tsp. salt
- 4 oz. shredded cheddar cheese

Directions:

1. Grease an 8x8-baking pan and preheat oven to 350 degrees F.
2. Slice each chili along the long side and open to where it lays flat.
3. Arrange half of the chilies on one side of the pan, skin side down in a single layer.
4. Top the chilies with pepper-jack cheese.
5. Put the remaining chilies on top of the cheese, skin side up.
6. Beat the eggs, cream, and salt well, and then pour over the chilies.
7. Top with cheddar cheese and bake in oven for 35 minutes or until golden brown.
8. Let it cool off for 12 minutes, serve and enjoy!

Number of servings: 9

Macros (per serving):

Calories: 211.0
Protein: 10.9 g
Carbs: 1.4 g
Fat: 17.6 g

*Recipe courtesy of THELMAGADDIS

Chapter 9: 15 High-Carb Recipes

Meat and Potatoes Dinner

Ingredients:

- 1 large potato
- 4 baby carrots
- 1/4 cup of onion
- 3 mushrooms
- Pat of butter
- 3 oz. extra lean ground beef
- Salt and pepper to taste

Directions:

1. Preheat oven to 450 degrees F.
2. Put a large piece of foil over a cookie sheet, spread butter over it, chop all of the vegetables (including potato), and put them on the sheet.
3. Put the hamburger chunks over the vegetables.
4. Roll the foil so the vegetables and beef stay inside.
5. Place the sheet in the oven and bake for 30 minutes.
6. Remove, let it cool and enjoy!

Number of servings: 1

Macros (per serving):

Calories: 564.1
Protein: 26.3 g
Carbs: 73.5 g

Fat: 19.4 g

*Recipe courtesy of RDEFASSI

Chocolate Chip Cookies

Ingredients:

- 2 1/2 cups white flour
- 3/4 cup granulated sugar
- 3 cups old fashioned Quaker oats
- 2 cups chopped walnuts
- 2 cups chocolate chips
- 2 sticks margarine butter
- 1 tsp. salt
- 1 tsp. baking soda
- 1 cup whey protein powder
- 1 tsp. vanilla flavoring
- 3 eggs

Directions:

1. Preheat oven to 350 degrees F
2. Cream the sugars and margarine butter.
3. Add in vanilla and eggs and beat until smooth.
4. Add in protein powder then salt, baking powder, and flour and mix until smooth.
5. Add in the chocolate chips, oatmeal and walnuts and stir until smooth.
6. Use a ¼ measuring cup to portion the dough and make each cookie roughly 3" in diameter and ½" high.
7. Bake for around 10 minutes until golden brown.
8. Let them sit and cool and enjoy!

Number of servings: 48

Macros (per serving):

Calories: 168.6
Protein: 6.5 g
Carbs: 18.8 g

Fat: 8.7 g

*Recipe courtesy of STIURF

Dinner Rolls

Ingredients:

- 1/4 cup honey
- 1 cup warm water
- 1 envelope yeast
- 1/3 cup non-fat dry milk
- 1/3 cup unsalted melted butter
- 2 eggs
- 1 tsp. salt
- 4 1/2 cups flour

Directions:

1. Dissolve honey and yeast in warm water and let it stand until foamy.
2. Add in the milk powder, butter, eggs and salt then stir.
3. Gradually add in the flour and knead for 8 minutes.
4. Let the dough rise until doubled in height, press them down again and let them rise for 30 minutes before putting them in the oven.
5. Form into 30 round rolls and place them on the baking sheet.
6. Bake in the oven at 375 degrees F for 15 minutes.
7. Let cool for 10 minutes, serve and enjoy!

Number of servings: 30

Macros (per serving):

Calories: 80.5
Protein: 2.3 g
Carbs: 14.8 g
Fat: 1.2 g

*Recipe courtesy of BKMNURSING

Ham and Green Bean Dinner

Ingredients:

- 2 lbs. quarter ham roast
- 6 medium sized potatoes
- 12 oz. can green beans
- 1 cup ginger ale

Directions:

1. Preheat oven to 450 degrees F.
2. Put ham roast on a baking pan and add one cup of ginger ale.
3. Place potatoes on separate pan and bake them at the same time as the ham roast.
4. Bake for about 35 minutes or until thoroughly cooked.
5. Boil the green beans while the ham roast and potatoes are baking on medium heat.
6. Serve and enjoy!

Number of servings: 6

Macros (per serving):

Calories: 190.7
Protein: 8.4 g
Carbs: 36.4 g
Fat: 1.5 g

*Recipe courtesy of NICOLE_SANTILLO

Salmon and Rice Dinner

Ingredients:

- 4 oz. wild salmon
- 1/2 cup whole grain brown rice
- 1 cup chopped broccoli
- 2 tsp. Parmesan grated cheese
- Sea salt to taste
- Garlic powder to taste
- Onion powder to taste
- Parsley to taste

Directions:

1. Preheat oven to broil.
2. Place salmon on non-stick pan with the scales facing down.
3. Season salmon with the sea salt, parsley, onion powder and garlic powder.
4. Bake the salmon for about 15 minutes.
5. While the salmon is baking, make the rice according to pkg. directions.
6. Then steam the broccoli until thoroughly heated.
7. When done, put the rice in a bowl and grate with Parmesan cheese.
8. Put rice on top of broccoli, remove the salmon and place on rice and enjoy!

Number of servings: 1

Macros (per serving):

Calories: 340.0
Protein: 29.0 g
Carbs: 32.0 g
Fat: 8.0 g
*Recipe courtesy of FAYETTESIDRA

Beef Hamburger

Ingredients:

- 6 oz. lean ground beef
- 1 hamburger bun
- 1 tbsp. light mayonnaise
- 1 tbsp. ketchup
- 1 tbsp. yellow mustard
- Toppings of your choosing

Directions:

1. Cook the ground beef on a skillet over medium heat until thoroughly cooked and there's no pink.
2. Toast the bun in a toaster.
3. Put 1 tbsp. of mayo on the bottom half of the bun.
4. Put the patty on the bottom half of the bun.
5. Add in the ketchup and mustard.
6. Put any additional toppings on the burger that you like.
7. Place the top bun on and enjoy!

Number of servings: 1

Macros (per serving):

Calories: 458.4
Protein: 38.9 g
Carbs: 26.9 g
Fat: 22.0 g

*Recipe courtesy of WHITEBOY23

Sausage and Black Beans

Ingredients:

- 1 tbsp. flour
- 2- 15 oz. cans black beans
- 2- 10 oz. packages frozen kernel corn
- 16 oz. jar chunky salsa
- 1 lb. smoked sliced sausage
- 1 cup Colby jack cheese

Directions:

1. Preheat oven to 450 degrees F.
2. In a large bowl, mix together the flour, beans, corn, salsa and sliced sausage.
3. Put the mixed ingredients in a large, extra heavy-duty foil bag in a 1-inch deep pan, arranged in an even layer.
4. Double fold the bag and seal it
5. Bake in the oven for 50-60 minutes.
6. Once done, hold the bag with mitts and cut it open with a knife.
7. Cautiously, fold back the top of the bag so the steam can escape.
8. Sprinkle with cheese, serve, and enjoy!

Number of servings: 5

Macros (per serving):

Calories: 546.4
Protein: 33.3 g
Carbs: 69.8 g
Fat: 14.9 g

*Recipe courtesy of CASSIDYR

Crockpot Turkey Dinner

Ingredients:

- 3/4 lb. turkey breast
- 1 can Campbell's cream of chicken soup
- 1/2 pkg. dry French onion soup mix
- 2 1/4 cup water
- 1 cup dry pearled barley
- 3 cups frozen green beans

Directions:

1. Put the turkey, soup mixes and 3/4 cup of water into the crockpot and cook on low for 6 hours.
2. After 6 hours have passed, add in the barley, remaining water and green beans, and continue cooking in the crockpot for an additional hour.
3. Serve and enjoy!

Number of servings: 6

Macros (per serving):

Calories: 328.0
Protein: 37.1 g
Carbs: 38.2 g
Fat: 2.5 g

*Recipe courtesy of GVMEMOMENT

Beef Spaghetti

Ingredients:

- 1 lb. lean ground beef
- 1/2 chopped onion
- 1/2 chopped green pepper
- 10 oz. drained canned mushrooms
- 28 oz. can diced tomatoes
- 8 oz. spaghetti, broken into 1-inch pieces
- 1 cup water
- 1 1/2 tsp. Italian seasoning
- Salt and pepper to taste

Directions:

1. In a large saucepan, brown the beef and onions over medium heat until the meat is no longer pink.
2. Throw in the green pepper and mushrooms and cook for a few more minutes.
3. Then add in the diced tomatoes, spaghetti and water and stir the mixture.
4. Add in the spices.
5. Cook and cover for 15 minutes, stirring occasionally or finish when spaghetti is tender.

Number of servings: 6

Macros (per serving):

Calories: 388.5
Protein: 21.1 g
Carbs: 38.7 g
Fat: 16.5 g

*Recipe courtesy of RAGGEDY_ANN

Calamari Salad

Ingredients:

For Salad:
- 3 cups tossed salad
- 1 large hardboiled egg, sliced in half
- 1/2 avocado
- 4 tbsp. shredded cheddar cheese
- 1 cubic inch crumbled feta cheese
- 8 pieces sun dried tomato

For Salad Garnish and Dressing:
- 2 lemon wedges
- 2 tsp. of olive oil
- Salt and pepper to taste

For Squid:
- 200 grams raw squid
- Salt and black pepper to taste
- 2 tsp. olive oil

Directions:

1. Slice the squid into rings, place in a bowl and drizzle with 2 tsp. of olive oil.
2. Add in salt and pepper, toss around to coat and let sit for 5 minutes.
3. Divide salad ingredients on two plates, using any other veggies you like.
4. Heat a skillet on medium heat and dump squid mixture onto skillet, sautéing for 7-10 minutes.
5. Divide squid on two plates and drizzle one tsp. of olive on each plate. Add salt and pepper and a lemon wedge to each and enjoy!

Number of servings: 2

Macros (per serving):

Calories: 418.5
Protein: 28.1 g
Carbs: 19.6 g
Fat: 26.6 g

*Recipe courtesy of KALEXIAS

Macaroni and Cheese Tuna Casserole

Ingredients:

- 1 box Kraft Mac N Cheese
- 1/4 cup skim milk
- 3 tsp. margarine
- 1 can tuna

Directions:

1. Boil the mac n cheese for about 8 minutes according to the box's instructions.
2. Drain the pasta.
3. Add in 1/4 cup of skim milk and stir.
4. Add in 3 tsp. of margarine and stir.
5. Add in the packet of cheese that comes with the macaroni and mix it in well.
6. Flake the tuna in the can with a fork and then add it to the macaroni and stir well.

Number of servings: 4

Macros (per serving):

Calories: 333.2
Protein: 27.6 g
Carbs: 39.8 g
Fat: 5.6 g

*Recipe courtesy of SUMMERRAINCITY

Tortellini & Bacon Dinner

Ingredients:

- 2 cups frozen tortellini
- 4 slices diced bacon
- 3 tbsp. chopped parsley
- 1 small yellow onion
- 1/2 cup Parmesan cheese
- Salt and pepper to taste

Directions:

1. Cook the frozen tortellini according to package directions and set to the side.
2. Cook the bacon until the pieces are golden brown.
3. Place the bacon bits on a paper towel to help drain the excess fat.
4. Cook the chopped onions on the same skillet used to cook the bacon until caramelized.
5. Put the bacon bits, tortellini and parsley back in and cook for another 3 minutes.
6. Next add in the Parmesan cheese and cook until it melts.
7. Serve and enjoy!

Number of servings: 4

Macros (per serving):

Calories: 230.3
Protein: 11.4 g
Carbs: 27.2 g
Fat: 8.4 g

*Recipe courtesy of MYLEHIA

Turkey Tenderloin Stir Fry

Ingredients:

- 8 oz. diced turkey cutlets
- 2 cups chopped Swiss chard
- 3 cloves garlic
- 1 medium onion
- 1 cup chopped green bell peppers
- 1 cup chopped mushrooms
- 1/2 cup chopped water chestnuts
- 1 cup chopped broccoli
- 3 tbsp. soy sauce
- 1/2 cup chicken broth
- 6 tsp. granulated sugar
- 2 tbsp. cornstarch
- 1 tbsp. peanut oil
- 3 tsp. ginger root

Directions:

1. Heat oil in pan and cook peppers and onions until lightly cooked.
2. Throw in the garlic and cook for a few additional minutes.
3. Cook the turkey tenderloins until golden brown.
4. Throw in the vegetables and sauté until lightly cooked.
5. Mix together the soy sauce, cornstarch, and chicken broth. Add this mixture to the stir-fry and cook until it slightly thickens.

Number of servings: 2

Macros (per serving):

Calories: 396.1
Protein: 34.5 g
Carbs: 51.1 g

Fat: 8.1 g

*Recipe courtesy of CSPEAKE

Venison Pot Roast

Ingredients:

- 2 1/2 lbs. venison
- 1/2 tsp. black pepper
- 1/4 tsp. salt
- 2 sliced large onions
- 1 3/4 cup water
- 1 packet onion soup mix
- 1 1/2 tbsp. balsamic vinegar
- 1 tsp. dried thyme
- 8 medium red potatoes
- 2 cups baby carrots

Directions:

1. Preheat oven to 350 degrees F.
2. Coat a pot with cooking spray and heat over medium heat.
3. Put the roast in the pan and sprinkle with salt and pepper and then place the onions around the roast.
4. Cook the roast and onions for roughly 8 minutes until they brown.
5. Add water into the pot and then stir in the soup mix, vinegar, and thyme and bring to a boil.
6. Move the roast and onions to a 9x13 pan and bake in the oven for 1 hour.
7. Put the potatoes and carrots around the roast, then cover and bake for another 2 hours until the vegetables are tender.
8. Finally, put the roast on a cutting board and slice it against the grain, then serve and enjoy!

Number of servings: 10

Macros (per serving):

Calories: 292.9
Protein: 29.4 g
Carbs: 33.0 g
Fat: 2.3 g

*Recipe courtesy of CASCHWARTZ620

Italian Sausage and Rice

Ingredients:

- 1- 6 oz. pkg. chicken rice
- 1 lb. bulk Italian sausage
- 1 cup chopped onion
- 1 clove minced garlic
- 1 cup water
- 1- 16 oz. can peeled whole tomatoes
- 1 tsp. basil leaves
- 2 cups chopped broccoli
- 1 cup grated mozzarella cheese
- 2 tbsp. chopped parsley

Directions:

1. Brown the sausage, onion and garlic in a large skillet.
2. Add in the water, tomatoes and basil, and bring to a boil.
3. Add in the rice, reduce the heat and simmer for 15 minutes.
4. Add the broccoli and cook for another 7-10 minutes until liquid is absorbed.
5. Remove the skillet from heat, and then sprinkle with mozzarella cheese and parsley.
6. Cover and let it sit for 5 minutes, and then serve and enjoy!

Number of servings: 48

Macros (per serving):

Calories: 599.8
Protein: 29.6 g
Carbs: 38.9 g
Fat: 36.3 g
*Recipe courtesy of JAMIECEE

Chapter 10: How to Track Your Calories and Macros

Tracking your calories and macros is imperative if you want to see success with carb cycling. This is going to be the most tedious part of the process, but it has to be done. If you don't measure how many carbs and calories you're consuming, you won't have a clue if you're actually eating low carbs on the days you're supposed to. Fortunately, there are some ways to make tracking your calories and macros easier.

The simplest and easiest way to track your calories and macronutrients is to go to the App Store or Google Play Store, type in macro tracker and download one of the many apps available. Any of the worthwhile apps will cost you a few dollars, but it'll pay for itself over and over again considering all of the time it'll save you. Once you download an app, all you have to do is type in the foods you eat. The app will then tell you how many calories the food has as well as its protein, carb and fat contents. The majority of the apps will even contain a handy bar code scanner, which will allow you to instantly scan and store calories and macros from whatever you eat.

The other thing that makes an app so useful is the fact that it's on your phone, which will be with you wherever you go. If you decide to go out to eat dinner, for example, you'll still be able to track your calories right then and there. Don't wait and tell yourself that you'll remember everything you ate. Track it as soon as possible for the best results!

Another item you'll want to invest in is a food scale. These are pretty cheap, and you can buy one on Amazon for about $11. A food scale will tell you the amount of grams or ounces that are in the foods you're eating. You can then use the formulas from the earlier chapters to calculate the number of calories in the food items. This will be very useful to be able to measure out serving sizes as closely as possible. For example, if a nutritional label says that one serving of steak is 32 grams, you'll have no way of knowing if you're actually eating 32 grams unless you measure it.

If you decide not to use your phone to track your macros then you'll have to measure everything by hand using a notebook, which can be extremely inconvenient. Tracking your calories in this manner will become a pain-in-the-neck rather quickly, and you'll give up on it entirely before too long. That's why I highly recommend you take the easy road and invest a couple of dollars in a macro app.

When it comes to tracking your calories and macros, it's important to be patient with yourself. You'll make mistakes at times, or you won't know the calories in a certain meal and that's ok. You have to stay calm and keep moving forward. When you get frustrated or rushed, you'll either quit or wrongly estimate how many calories are in what you're eating. And unfortunately, if you're not able to be diligent with tracking your calories and macros, you won't be successful with carb cycling.

The cool thing is that after a while, you'll get a good feel for how to you need to eat during your high and low carb days. You'll know approximately how much calories and macros are in the meals you're regularly eating. You can simply eyeball it and take an accurate guess as to how many calories are in the foods you're eating.

Of course this is something you'll acquire as time goes on with practice, so again remember that patience is the key! Initially though, tracking your macros can be frustrating at times if you've never done it before, so use the first couple of weeks as practice and a learning experience. The good news is that you don't need to be totally accurate down to the exact calorie when measuring. For example, if you need to eat 150 grams of protein one day, it's unlikely that you'll actually eat 150 grams spot on. That's completely ok; you want to get as close as you can, but don't go crazy trying to hit the numbers exactly. You want to largely be accurate and consistent for the long haul.

Chapter 11 Frequently Asked Questions

Can I Treat My High-Carb Days Like a Cheat Day?

No, you can't. There's a difference between a high-carb day and a cheat day. A cheat day brings with it the mentality that you can eat whatever you want whenever you want. This can make things get out of hand at times, causing you to overeat. A high-carb day, on the other hand, is a strategic part of the carb cycling process. You're still limited to eating a moderate amount of fat, and you'll want the majority of your carbs to come from quality food sources.

What if I'm not losing or gaining weight eating 13 calories per pound of bodyweight?

If you've been struggling to lose weight eating 13 calories per pound of bodyweight then I recommend using a different method to set your calories. Before I get into that though, you must first make sure you were actually eating 13 calories per pound of bodyweight minus 500 calories to lose 1 pound per week. It's easy to overestimate the amount of calories you're eating, and this could be the reason why you're not seeing results.

Once you've made sure you've accurately been tracking your calories, you can take your goal bodyweight, multiply it by 11 and then eat that many calories (don't subtract anything from the final calculated number).

Yes, I understand that your goal bodyweight will be a random number that you think you'll look good at, so take your best guess. Start on the higher side and work your way down from there if you still aren't losing weight.

    Here's an example for a 250-pound male.

    Current Weight 250

    Goal Bodyweight 200

    200 x 11= 2,200 daily calories

    Let's say once this person reaches his goal of 200 pounds, he's still not satisfied with how he looks. From there, he can simply set a new goal bodyweight (i.e. 190 pounds for example) and go from there.

On the other hand, let's say you're struggling to add muscle eating 13 calories per pound of bodyweight plus 250 calories. Again, make sure you're accurately tracking the amount of calories you're eating. You could be miscounting your calories, and that would account for why you're not gaining any weight. Once you've made sure you're tracking things accurately, you can add 100 calories to your total resting metabolic rate weekly until you start gaining weight. For example:

A 180-pound male looking to gain weight would multiply his bodyweight by 13 to determine his maintenance calories.

180 x 13= 2,340

This person would then add 250 calories to 2,340 and get a total of 2,590 calories per day. If he eats 2,590 calories on a daily basis, he should start to gain 0.5 pound per week. However, if he doesn't, he can simply add 100 calories to his original 2,590 calories on a weekly basis until he does.

For example, on week 1, he would eat 2,690 calories. If he didn't gain any weight by the end of the week, he would eat 2,790 calories for the following week, and so on and so forth until he starts gaining weight.

What if I hit a plateau and I stop losing weight at my regular pace?

Let's say you've been losing weight just fine, but then all of the sudden you hit a wall and stop losing weight. In this case, take your new current bodyweight (which should be a lower number from when you first started) and multiply that by 13.

Take that number and subtract 250 from it. This will be your new daily caloric intake for you to lose weight.

This will have you losing weight at a rate of approximately 0.5 pound per week. You may have previously been losing weight at a rate of 1 pound per week, but now you'll lose at a rate of 0.5 pound per week.

This is because I don't want you to drastically reduce your calories all of the sudden, and because if you've hit a plateau, you're likely very close to hitting your goal weight anyway.

How many meals should I eat per day?

You can eat as many meals as you like throughout the day. Meal frequency doesn't matter for weight loss (16), but the total amount of calories you eat does. So eat however is easiest for you and your schedule.

I, myself, prefer to eat 3 meals a day and that works great for most people. However, feel free to eat 6 times per day or even as little as once per day. As long as you're hitting your macros, you'll be fine.

What do I do once I reach my goal bodyweight?

Contrary to what you might be thinking, things aren't going to be that much different from what you've been doing to lose weight. You still need to do flexible dieting and continue eating in the same manner that you previously were. This means that you should still keep the same eating schedule and keep eating similar meals to the ones that you were eating to lose weight.

However, there's one difference between maintenance and creating a caloric deficit to lose weight. The difference is that you get to consume more calories! How many calories? Well, this is pretty easy to figure out as a matter of fact.

Step #1: Determine at what rate you were losing weight (i.e. 1 pound per week).

Step #2: Translate pounds lost per week into calories.
      0.5 pound lost per week= 250 calories
      1 pound lost per week= 500 calories
      1.5 pounds lost per week= 750 calories
      2 pounds lost per week= 1,000 calories, etc.

Step #3: Add in those additional calories to what you were previously eating to maintain your new weight.

For example, let's say someone was losing weight at a rate of 1 pound per week by eating 1,850 calories per day. Once he hits his goal weight, he needs to eat 2,350 calories (1,850+500) per day to maintain his new weight.

You'll also need to recalculate your macro percentages. Continuing with this example, this individual would need to do the following with his new caloric intake:

2,350 x .40= 940 daily calories from protein
2,350 x .35= 822.5 daily calories from carbs

2,350 x .25= 587.5 daily calories from fat

How much weight should I lift during the workouts?

Lift as much weight as you possibly can for the given rep range. Initially, you won't know how much weight to use, so you'll have to take your best guess. For example, let's say you're doing bench press for 8 reps. You think you can lift around 150 pounds for that many reps, but on your first set, you easily complete 10 reps.

This means the weight is too light and you need to increase it for the next set. On the next set, you lift 165 pounds and struggle to complete the 8th rep. This is what you want to happen, and it means you've found a good weight to use. Once you can complete all 3 sets for 8 reps with 165 pounds, move up to 170 the next time you bench press. If you can't complete 8 reps for all 3 sets, stick with 165 until you can. Here's an example:

Workout 1: Bench Press with 165 pounds
Set 1: 8 reps
Set 2: 8 reps
Set 3: 7 reps

Because you only completed 7 reps on the last set, stick with 165 for the next workout.

Workout 2: Bench Press with 165 pounds
Set 1: 8 reps
Set 2: 8 reps
Set 3: 8 reps

Because you completed all 3 sets for 8 reps, move up to 170 on your next workout with bench press.

Note: It's better to use a weight that's too heavy and miss a rep or two than it is to use a weight that's too light and leave some reps in the tank. For example, it's better to do 170 pounds and only complete 6 reps instead of 8 as opposed to using 155 pounds and stopping at 8 reps even though you could've easily done more reps.

How Fast Should I Lose Weight?

The more weight you have to lose, the faster the rate at which you can lose the weight. For example, if you have 50+ pounds to lose, you can lose weight at a rate of 2 pounds or more per week. If you only have 5 pounds to lose, then lose weight at a rate of 0.5 pound per week.

For most people, losing 1 pound per week is the sweet spot. You'll be creating an average caloric deficit of 500 calories daily. At this pace, you'll be losing weight fairly quickly, and you won't be miserable all of the time from a complete lack of calories.

How much water should I drink on a daily basis?

Your body is made up of about 60% water, so it's important to consume water for several reasons. Drinking water regularly:

- Helps keep your joints and ligaments fluid, which can help prevent injury
- Helps control your caloric intake
- Flushes out toxins
- Improves skin quality
- Improves kidney function
- Improves your focus

Many people recommend that you should drink 1 gallon of water per day. This is a blanket answer that doesn't meet individual needs. This recommendation would have a 100-pound woman drinking the same amount of water as a 200-pound man. Absurd!

Other health experts advise drinking eight 8-ounce glasses (64 ounces total) of water a day. But again 64 ounces isn't going to be enough for most people. What should you do then? I don't keep track of my water intake—I go by how I feel and the color of my urine.

Your body's own thirst mechanism will be accurate in telling you if you need more water. If you feel thirsty, go drink some water. If not, you're probably ok. You can also use the color of your urine to judge how hydrated you are. If your urine is yellow, then you should drink more water. If it's clear then you should be good to go. This keeps things simple and it's one less thing you have to keep track of.

Are there any supplements that you recommend I take?

Most supplements are a complete waste of money. There's not a single supplement that's required in order for you to build muscle or burn fat. In fact, I advise for the first 6 weeks of your IIFYM diet that you don't take *any* supplements at all.

This is because I want you to see for yourself that it really is possible for you to get results without supplements. Your hard work and dedication matter way more than any pill or powder.

With that being said, there are a few supplements I recommend if you have the budget for them:

#1: Protein Powder:

You can't have a recommended list of supplements without protein powder on the list, right? Just kidding. But this has to be one of the most overhyped supplements of all time.

I think that the media does a really good job of making us believe that we must take protein powder to build muscle or take it to prevent muscle loss. I do think that protein powder can provide some benefits if *you need it.*

If you struggle to consistently hit your macros with protein then I would consider investing in a protein powder. Protein is necessary to help build and prevent the breakdown of muscle.

Therefore, ensuring that your muscle is spared is a good thing. However, don't go out of your way and eat more calories just for the sake of consuming more protein.

#2: Fish/Krill Oil

These oils are great sources of Omega-3 fatty acids. This is a good thing because most people consume too many Omega-6 fatty acids with foods like vegetable and canola oil.

Ideally, you want to be consuming a 1 to 1 ratio of Omega-3's to Omega-6's. Fish and krill oil can help you narrow the gap between the two types of fatty acids that you're consuming.

The main benefit from consuming these oils is that they act as an anti-inflammatory in your body. When you consume Omega-6's on the other hand, they act as an inflammatory.

That's why it's important to strike a balance with both of the fatty acids. The anti-inflammatory benefit is great because it can reduce your risk of developing heart disease or high blood pressure.

Finally, reducing inflammation can aid in muscle recovery. If you're going to invest in fish or krill oil, make sure that it's a very high-grade supplement.

The way that some of the lower quality oils are processed inhibits the absorption of them, which would make them completely useless. As for investing in fish or krill oil, taking either one is fine really.

Krill oil does contain the antioxidant astaxanthin (17), which helps with joint health, boosts cognitive function and helps promote a healthy cholesterol balance, while fish oil does not. However, I have noticed that krill oil can be harder to find, and it's typically more expensive so don't sweat not buying it.

#3: Digestive Enzymes

This is my favorite supplement of all time, and it's probably one of the most underrated supplements as well. If your body can't absorb the vitamins and nutrients that you're consuming then what's the point?

The sad fact of the matter is that when our foods get cooked, many of the enzymes get destroyed. Digestive enzymes will not only help to replenish those enzymes missed from cooked foods, but it will also help your body to better break down and utilize the nutrients that you're eating.

Also, if you ever suffer regularly from bloating, heartburn or have bad skin, give digestive enzymes a try and see if you notice a difference. Of course, it's important to note that these enzymes need to be high quality if you want them to be of any use.

Simply going to the local grocery store and purchasing a $10 bottle of enzymes isn't going to cut it. You must buy a high-quality enzyme if you want to get any use out of it. Personally, I recommend using Bio Trust.

How Do I Motivate Myself to Go to the Gym?

Finding the motivation to go to the gym or eat right can be hard. No matter who you are, there will be times when you don't feel like working out. Having that feeling is ok, but you can't let it control you. There will be times when you'll have to do it anyway even when you don't feel like it.

That's what will ultimately separate a long-term successful fitness journey from failing at it. I do have some tips to help you out along the way:

Tip #1: Focus on Gradual Improvements

Many people make fitness an all-or-nothing game. They tell themselves that they'll workout 5 days a week and eat clean 100% of the time for the rest of their lives. Let's say you workout only 4 days one week. Are you a failure?

Of course not! You still worked out 4 days, but in your mind you are because you failed to reach 5 workouts. You make it hard to celebrate any small successes that you do have because the standards are too high.

Instead, focus on making smaller, more gradual improvements and celebrate any successes you have along the way. For example, start off with a goal to only workout 2 days per week if it's been years since you've last worked out. Once you achieve that goal, you'll feel good about yourself then you can move up to working out 3 days per week and so on.

Tip #2: Action Leads Motivation

People think they have to get the inspiration or motivation from somewhere in order to take the action necessary to workout. The reverse of that is actually true. You need to start by taking an action no matter how small. And once you get started, you'll likely want to continue on with what you're doing.

When I think about everything I have to do to workout such as put my gym clothes on, drive to the gym, workout with a bunch of grueling exercises, drive back and shower, I start to make up silly excuses as to why I should skip this time.

Instead, I'll tell myself to do just one exercise when I get to the gym and not pressure myself to do anything more. After I finish that first exercise, it's always easier for me to finish the rest of the workout.

You just have to get started. Try this out for any healthy habit you want to start. For example, if you want to start flossing your teeth, tell yourself you'll only floss one tooth and don't pressure yourself to do anything more than that!

Tip #3: Put Your Own Money on the Line

Money is a very powerful motivator. And you can use your own money to motivate yourself to start working out more. Here's what you're going to do—give someone a good amount of money. Not $20, but something that would actually hurt you—$100, $200, $500, or whatever you can't afford to lose.

Then tell your friend that if you don't go to the gym 3 days this week, for example, they get to keep the money. When you give up the money in the first place, you'll fight to get it back. This is much different than telling yourself you'll give the money to someone after you miss your workouts.

It's too easy to make an excuse and not give away the money. Give the money up in the first place and make sure your friend actually holds you accountable to it. This is by far the best way to get motivation to workout. There's a real cost involved if you don't comply. You'll either get ripped or go broke trying.

Conclusion

Thanks for getting this book and reading it all the way through to the end! Carb cycling is a good way to get and stay in shape for the rest of your life. You simply have to stay dedicated. Carb cycling works as long as you put forth the effort needed.

Feel free to email me at thomas@rohmerfitness.com with any fitness questions you may have.

And finally, if this book was helpful, please take a few minutes and leave a review. Your feedback will help me make better content for you in the future!

Sources

(1) https://www.ncbi.nlm.nih.gov/pubmed/8697046

(2) http://ajcn.nutrition.org/content/early/2013/06/26/ajcn.113.064113.abstract

(3) https://www.ncbi.nlm.nih.gov/pmc/articles/PMC3419346/

(4) https://www.ncbi.nlm.nih.gov/pubmed/16918875

(5) https://www.ncbi.nlm.nih.gov/pubmed/16320856

(6) http://circ.ahajournals.org/content/106/4/523.full

(7) https://www.hindawi.com/journals/isrn/2013/435027/

(8) https://www.ncbi.nlm.nih.gov/pubmed/19927027

(9) https://www.ncbi.nlm.nih.gov/pmc/articles/PMC4213385/

(10) https://www.ncbi.nlm.nih.gov/pubmed/19935843

(11) https://www.ncbi.nlm.nih.gov/pmc/articles/PMC3381813/

(12) http://www.ncbi.nlm.nih.gov/pubmed/18197184

(13) http://www.ncbi.nlm.nih.gov/pubmed/20473222

(14) http://www.health.harvard.edu/newsletter_article/Walking-Your-steps-to-health

(15) https://www.ncbi.nlm.nih.gov/pubmed/18787373

*Recipes courtesy of users at sparkpeople.com

DASH Diet

Overcome Hypertension, Lose Weight, and Experience a New Level of Health

Thomas Rohmer

Copyright © 2018
Rohmerfitness All rights reserved.

No part of this publication may be reproduced, distributed, or
transmitted in any form or by any means, including photocopying, recording, or other electronic or mechanical methods, without the prior written permission and consent of the publisher, except in the in the case of brief quotations embodied in product reviews and certain other non-commercial uses permitted by copyright law.

Disclaimer:

This guide has been created for informational and reference purposes only. The author, publisher, and any other affiliated parties cannot be held in any way accountable for any personal injuries or damage allegedly resulting from the information contained herein, or from any misuse of such guidance. Although strict measures have been taken to provide accurate information, the parties involved with the creation and publication of this guide take no responsibility for any issues that many arise from alleged discrepancies contained herein. It is strongly recommended that you consult a physician, personal trainer, and nutritionist prior to commencing this or any other workout or diet plan. This guide is not a substitute for professional personal guidance from a qualified medical professional. If you feel pain or discomfort at any point during exercises contained herein, cease the activity immediately and seek medical guidance.

Table of Contents

Chapter 1: What is the DASH Diet?......................246
Chapter 2: Best Foods to Eat on the DASH Diet..248
Chapter 3: Foods You'll Want to Limit on the DASH Diet..259
Chapter 4: Health Benefits of the DASH Diet......268
Chapter 5: How to Easily Follow the DASH Diet for a Long Time to Come...277
Chapter 6: What Kind of Exercise Works Best with the DASH Diet?...282
Chapter 7: Setting Up and Starting Your DASH Diet Plan..289
Chapter 8: 14-Day DASH Diet Sample Meal Plan..299
Chapter 9: Frequently Asked Questions...............316

Introduction:

It's the 21st century and we've made great advances in things like technology and medicine. However, when it comes to our health, we seem to have taken a step back. People today are ridden with things like Type 2 Diabetes and cardiovascular disease among other things. Why is it that we've made such great improvements in certain areas like technology, yet the obesity rate continues to increase?

It comes down to the wrong information. We are constantly being sold on gimmicks like weight loss pills and other sketchy powders and potions that are supposed to magically help us lose weight, get our blood pressure in check, and make us healthy again. But clearly none of those things are coming true. We try diet after diet in the hopes that it'll finally be the answer, and all we end up with is disappointment.

Luckily this all changes for you today. In this book, you'll discover what has been named as the best diet multiple years in a row. It's not some gimmicky overnight fix. Instead it's something that actually works.

I'm talking about the DASH diet here. This nutritional approach will finally allow you to lose weight and get your health back. Not only that, but it isn't that hard of a diet to follow! Most diets have confusing rules like you can only eat at a certain time or they force you to eat certain foods.

That won't be the case with the DASH diet. In this book, you'll learn about all of the ins and outs of the DASH diet. You'll understand all of the health benefits you can expect to gain from following this eating plan. You'll even learn how to use exercise to further benefit your nutrition plan. And finally you'll be given a step-by-step process along with a 14-day sample meal plan to help you get started on the right foot with the DASH diet. Let's dive in and get started...

Chapter 1: What is the DASH Diet?

The DASH diet stands for dietary approaches to stop hypertension, and the main goal of the diet is to do just that—stop hypertension. Hypertension is high blood pressure, and it's something that affects more people than you might think. According to the CDC, high blood pressure affects nearly 75 million American adults (1). That's nearly 1 out of every 3 people!

And of the people who do have high blood pressure, approximately half of those people don't have it under control (2)! You might be wondering why having high blood pressure is such a big deal. Hypertension can lead to heart and kidney disease, stroke, and even blindness.

And with the way most people eat, it starts to become much more apparent as to why our blood pressure is getting out of control. The standard American diet (which stands for SAD) consists mostly of processed foods, artificially sweetened foods, red meats, foods high in salt, and take out food at least once per week, but possibly more often than that (3).

In addition to that, 1 out of every 3 Americans are either overweight or obese (4), and show signs of metabolic syndrome. Metabolic syndrome is characterized by having excess weight, especially around the stomach/abdomen area, high blood pressure, slightly higher blood sugar, and problems with cholesterol and the number of triglycerides in the blood.

So clearly something needs to change in regards to the way that most people are eating nowadays. The DASH diet cannot only help you lower your blood pressure, but it can also help you maintain a healthy bodyweight. The primary focus of the DASH diet is to help you eat the right amount of fruits, vegetables, whole grains, and low-fat dairy products.

These types of foods are high in fiber, contain a moderate amount of fat, and are rich in potassium, calcium, and magnesium. Consuming more of these nutrients and minerals will help you to start seeing some improvements in your overall health by doing things like lowering blood pressure, improving digestion, and staying fuller for a longer period of time.

The DASH diet also will reduce salt intake, saturated fat, processed foods, eliminate trans fat, and sweets. With the DASH diet eating plan, it's not just about what foods you're going to be consuming. Equally as important are what foods you're going to drastically reduce or eliminate altogether.

You can eat all of the nutrient-rich foods that you want such as fruits and vegetables, and that's great! However, the thing you have to remember is that you can quickly offset the benefits of those healthy foods by eating junk. Consuming processed foods, salty foods, or foods that aren't that healthy will do you no good and cause you to take a step back in your quest to become a healthier individual.

So don't think of this diet strictly in terms of what you'll be eating because what you eliminate from your diet will be equally as important to your success with the diet plan.

Chapter 2: Best Foods to Eat on the DASH Diet

The following are the best foods you can eat while on the DASH diet. These are foods that are high in fiber, magnesium, potassium, and other vitamins and minerals. This is not meant to be a comprehensive list, rather this is meant to give you some good ideas for what you should be eating while on the DASH diet.

Vegetables

While following the DASH diet, you should be consuming around 4-5 servings of vegetables per day. We all know that vegetables are good for us and that they are very healthy foods, yet I think few of us realize just how healthy vegetables really are:

- Eating vegetables regularly can help to reduce the risk of heart disease and stroke (5).

- It can help protect you against certain types of cancer (6).

- Vegetables are low in calories and high in fiber. This means that you can eat as much of them as you want and not have to worry about overeating. And the fiber will help to keep you fuller for a longer period of time as well as ensure proper bowel movements.

- Vegetables are very nutrient dense, meaning that they contain a lot of nutrients even though they're low in overall calories. Something like a candy bar, on the other hand, isn't nutrient dense. It contains a lot of calories, but it has very few nutrients.

- Folic acid: folic acid helps the body to create red blood cells. Red blood cells are necessary for transporting oxygen throughout your body. Getting proper amounts of folic acid is especially important for pregnant women or women who plan on becoming pregnant to ensure proper fetal development.

- Vegetables are rich in so many vitamins and minerals! Vegetables contain high amounts of vitamin A, C, potassium, iron, magnesium, and calcium.

Here's a list of vegetables that you should consume on the DASH diet:

- Sweet potatoes
- Tomatoes
- Squash
- Spinach
- Potatoes
- Lima Beans
- Kale
- Green Beans
- Peas
- Collard Greens
- Mustard Greens
- Broccoli
- Cauliflower
- Carrots

Fruits

Just like vegetables, fruits are very good for you and will provide you with many of the same vitamins and minerals that vegetables will. Unfortunately, fruits sometimes get a bad reputation because they contain fructose, which is a type of sugar. The thing is though that fructose is a natural sugar, not a processed sugar, and the benefits you'll receive from eating fruits far outweighs the fact that they contain some sugar in them.

While following the DASH diet eating plan, you'll want to consume 4-5 servings of fruit per day. Here are some of the amazing benefits of eating fruit:

- Fruits contain low amounts of sodium, calories, and fat.

- Similar to vegetables, fruit is very nutrient dense. So basically you'll be getting a good bang-for-your-buck when it comes to getting the most nutrients for the least amount of calories. Eating rich nutrient dense foods is critical for your success with the DASH diet.

- Fruits can help to lower cholesterol levels as well as reduce the risk for heart disease (7).

- Additionally, fruits contain high amounts of vitamin A and C, potassium, magnesium, folic acid, and fiber.

- Fruits also contain high amounts of water, which will help to keep your body hydrated.

Here's a list of fruits you should consume on the DASH diet:

- Raisins
- Blueberries
- Raspberries
- Strawberries
- Peaches
- Pineapples
- Melons

- Grapes
- Apples
- Apricots
- Bananas
- Dates
- Oranges
- Grapefruit
- Mangoes
- Tangerines

Dairy

While on the DASH diet eating plan, you should be consuming around 2-3 servings of dairy per day. It's important to note that you'll want to be eating low-fat dairy. The DASH diet limits certain types of fat intake, and consuming large amounts of fat through dairy isn't ideal, especially if it can be avoided in the first place. Here are some of the key benefits of consuming dairy in your diet:

- Dairy is high in protein. Protein is one of three macronutrients (carbs and fat being the other two), and it's responsible for aiding in many of your body's functions. One of the main things protein does is rebuild and repair tissue.

  It's an important building block for muscle, bone, skin, cartilage, and blood. It's also needed for the growth of hair and nails. So needless to say, protein is a very critical nutrient regardless if you're looking to pack on muscle or not.

- Dairy is rich in calcium. When you think of strong bones, what do you think of? You probably think of some kid or adult drinking a glass of milk. We've really been bombarded with the fact that milk (and other dairy products for that matter) is good for strong bones, and it really is so true! This is all because of calcium. Calcium is necessary for maintaining bone mass in the body, which helps to support the skeleton.

The thing is though we lose a lot of calcium through normal bodily processes in the kidneys and colon. Calcium is also used in muscle and nerve functions as well. And if we don't supply our bodies with enough calcium, then our bodies will start to pull the stored calcium in our bones in order to carry out its normal everyday functions.

This is why it's so important to be able to get the proper amount of calcium. It's not just used for our bones, but for many other necessary functions of our bodies. If we're not consuming an adequate amount of calcium, then that's when our bones will take a hit.

They'll start to become more brittle and frail. This can then lead to osteoporosis. Approximately 44 million Americans suffer from osteoporosis or low bone mass, and 55% of Americans over the age of 50 have osteoporosis (8). Osteoporosis will lead to more bone and hip fractures, which will inhibit mobility along with making it much harder to follow a diet plan such as DASH.

The following are some good sources of dairy that you can eat. Remember to go with the low-fat option when possible:

- Skim Milk
- 1% Milk
- Low-Fat Cheese
- Low-Fat Cottage Cheese
- Low-Fat Yogurt

Meats, Poultry, and Fish

You'll also be consuming some meat on the DASH diet plan. Meat isn't as heavily emphasized as some of the other food groups, such as fruits and vegetables however, it's still an important part of the diet regime. You'll want to consume around 1-2 servings of meat, poultry, and/or fish per day.

When consuming these meats, you'll want to make sure that you're going with lean meats. Additionally, be sure to trim away any visible fat from the meat that you can. Finally, the way you cook and prepare the meat matters as well. Avoid frying the food as this will make it have excess fat that isn't necessary. Instead, you'll want to broil, roast, or poach the meat.

This is the healthiest way to prepare your food. On a side note, when you're preparing poultry, remove the skin. Getting rid of the skin will help to remove more of the fat content contained in the chicken. Here are some of the benefits of consuming meat, poultry, and fish:

- High in protein: Similar to dairy products, any meat that you consume will have a good amount of protein in it. As mentioned earlier, this is important for repairing muscle tissue, growing hair and nails, as well as being an important building block for skin, bone, cartilage, and blood.

- Lean meats also contain a high amount of magnesium. Magnesium is critical for the proper functioning of hundreds of enzymes. Research has shown that magnesium can help to reduce blood pressure with individuals who are suffering from hypertension (9).

  It can also help with type 2 diabetes (10). And it can even help to fight depression (11). Fortunately, the DASH diet will allow you to consume plenty of magnesium, not just from lean meats, but from other food sources as well. Here's a list of lean meats that you can consume:

- Poultry
- Fish
- Bison
- Venison
- Beef

Nuts, Seeds, and Dried Beans

You'll want to consume 3 servings of various nuts, seeds, and dried beans per week on the DASH diet. You'll be eating quite a bit less of this food group compared to some of the other food groups, and it's for a good reason. Nuts are comprised mostly of fat.

Yes, there are good types of fat and bad types of fat (more on this later), however fat contains 9 calories per gram. On the other hand, protein and carbs only contain 4 calories per gram of food. This means that you'll be consuming over twice the amount of calories for the same amount of food if you're consuming fat. Those calories can add up rather quickly, and this is something we want to be aware of.

That's why you'll only be consuming 3 servings per week of these different nuts, seeds, and dried beans. As I just mentioned though, there is such a thing as good fat and bad fat. Bad fats would be something like trans fat and saturated fat. Excessive amounts of these types of fat have been shown to increase the risk for heart disease as well as other health problems (12).

Nuts and seeds, on the other hand, contain mono and polyunsaturated fats. These are a healthy type of fat that can help to lower your risk of heart disease by decreasing your low-density lipoproteins (LDL) and maintaining your high-density lipoproteins (HDL). Your LDL's are the bad type of cholesterol, and your HDL's are the good kind of cholesterol.

Of course, this idea of there being a good type of fat might be hard for you to grasp at first. Just like myself, you probably grew up learning that fat is bad for you. Intuitively this makes sense because we can see how excess fat on our bodies is bad for us so it naturally makes sense that consuming fat is harmful. However, this couldn't be further from the truth.

The reality is that consuming too many calories overall from all three macronutrients (protein, carbs, and fat) is bad for us and that's what leads to weight gain. Yes, certain types of fat should be limited or avoided altogether (such as saturated or trans fat), but that's not to say that all fat is bad for you because that simply isn't the case. Here are some of the benefits of consuming nuts, seeds, and dried beans:

- They are a rich source of energy. As I talked about earlier, fat contains 9 calories per gram. This can be dangerous if overeaten, however you have to remember why we're eating food in the first place—to get energy! Our body needs daily energy to maintain itself and carry out its daily functions.

  And where do our bodies get that needed energy? It gets it from the foods that we eat of course! Eating nuts is a great way to give our bodies a solid source of calories if we need to consume more. Just be careful not to overdo it!

- Contain healthy amounts of magnesium and fiber. Are you starting to notice a common theme here? Many of the foods you'll be consuming on the DASH diet are rich in magnesium! It's such a key mineral for getting and staying healthy, especially if you have hypertension.

Not only that, but nuts, seeds, and dried beans contain fiber. This is something that the typical American doesn't get enough of, and it's no wonder why so many people struggle with digestive issues.

- Finally, this food group surprisingly contains a good amount of protein. This is something you might not expect at first, but it's certainly true. For example, one serving of almonds contains 6 grams of protein! So not only will you be consuming healthy fats when you eat nuts, but you'll also be getting a decent amount of protein as well.

Now that you know the benefits of this food group, here's a list of some different kinds of them you can eat on the DASH diet (of course always go with the unsalted version whenever possible):

- Almonds
- Hazelnuts
- Mixed Nuts
- Peanuts
- Walnuts
- Sunflower Seeds
- Natural Peanut Butter
- Natural Almond Butter
- Kidney Beans
- Lentils
- Split Peas

Fats and Oils

Fats and oils are another essential part of the DASH diet. Again fats have gotten a bad reputation over the years, but it isn't all justified. The same goes for oils. When you think of oily food, what do you typically think of? Probably something that's greasy, fried, contains a lot of fat, and is unhealthy for you right?

Well yes, some oils are really bad for you. However, not all oils are as bad as they might seem. As I mentioned earlier, there are good fats and bad fats. You want to limit bad fats from your diet such as saturated fat and trans fat.

And you'll want to consume more healthy fats like mono and polyunsaturated fats. That's why you'll want to use oils that contain healthy fats like mono and polyunsaturated fats. The best kind of oil you can use for is olive oil. This is a healthy type of oil that contains a good amount of monounsaturated fat.

Canola oil can be a good option to use as well due to its high monounsaturated fat content as well, but use olive oil when you can as a first option. In terms of how much fats and oils you should be consuming, look to get roughly 2 servings of fats and oils per day. Here are some of the benefits of consuming fats and oils:

- Regulation of body temperature: Fats are important for regulating your body temperature and helping to keep it at a normal and healthy range.

- Good for brain health: non-water soluble vitamins such as vitamins A, D, E, and K need fat to get absorbed and transported by the body. These vitamins are critical for a properly functioning brain. Not only that, but your brain is made up of close to 60% fat (13)! So needless to say, it's quite important that you get an adequate amount of fat in your diet.

- Source of energy: fat can be stored in the body for later use, however it can also be used as a more primary source of energy if the body is low on carbohydrates or low on calories.

- Healthy skin and hair: Fat can help to make skin and hair appear soft, silky, and smooth due to its protective qualities. Without this protection from fat, harmful chemicals would be able to more easily enter the body through the skin.

Whole Grains

On the DASH eating plan, you're going to want to consume 6-8 servings of whole grains per day. It's very important to note that you'll want to be consuming whole grains here and not refined grains. Refined grains are more processed than whole grains and thus lose vitamins, minerals, and fiber during the process.

Whole grains, on the other hand, contain more vitamins and fiber, which is key to keeping you fuller longer. Whole grains still contain all three parts of the grain, which are the bran, germ, and endosperm.

When refined grains get processed, they're stripped of the bran and germ, which contain many key nutrients. Not only that, but whole grains are rich in things such as thiamin, riboflavin, niacin, and folate. These are part of the B vitamins complex. B vitamins are important for many different things including:

- Making new cells
- Red cell production
- Increase in HDL cholesterol (which is the good kind of cholesterol)
- Preventing memory loss
- Keeping depression at bay

Here's a list of acceptable whole grains should you eat while on the DASH diet:

- Whole-wheat pasta
- Whole-wheat bread
- Brown rice
- Whole-grain cereal

Chapter 3: Foods You'll Want to Limit on the DASH Diet

One of the things I really like about the DASH diet is that it doesn't entirely forbid you to eat the foods you love. I've seen plenty of people start a new diet plan only to fail a few short weeks later when they couldn't handle the misery anymore. Here's how it usually goes down:

1. You start a new diet and get all excited about it.
2. You immediately go cold turkey and cut all junk food from your diet.
3. For the first few days and maybe even weeks, things go pretty smoothly.
4. Then something comes up, like your best friend's birthday party for example.
5. While at the party, you do your best to stay on track with your diet plan.
6. You see everyone around you having a good time and eating as they please.
7. You really can't handle it anymore so you tell yourself you've been good and one piece of cake can't hurt that bad right?
8. You eat the piece of cake and then proceed to binge eat everything in sight.
9. Later that night you feel guilty for binge eating junk food and feel disgusted with yourself.
10. You also wonder if you'll ever be able to get the hang of this diet thing.
11. Then a few days or weeks later when you're feeling better about yourself, you start a new diet and the cycle repeats itself.

You see the problem in the above scenario isn't the fact that the person ate a slice of birthday cake. The reality is that one piece of cake, one brownie, one bowl of ice cream, etc. *can't* completely wreck your diet in one fell swoop. What does ruin your diet is when you feel guilty for eating something you feel like you shouldn't of.

These feelings of guilt then cause you to say "screw it," which is when you'll proceed to binge eat anything your heart desires at that moment. And it's the binge eating that'll mess up your nutrition plan. Instead, a much better approach is to occasionally allow sweets or other treats in your diet from time to time.

Think about it, if it's in your diet plan to eat a small bowl of ice cream every three days, are you going to feel guilty when you eat that ice cream? No, you won't because it's part of the diet plan! On the flip side, if all junk food is forbidden under any circumstances, how are you going to feel if you eat a sweet treat? You'll feel horrible!

You'll feel like you cheated on your diet and that it's all over with. That, of course, isn't true, but at that moment, most people feel like complete failures. And this is one of the things I love most about the DASH diet. On the DASH diet eating plan, you're allowed to eat up to five servings of sweets per week.

This means that you won't have to completely give up your favorite sweet treats if you don't want to. The DASH diet is realistic about the fact that we're human. Seriously, who do you know of that could go the rest of their lives without eating another piece of junk food ever again? Probably no one! That's why the DASH diet is really not a diet as much as it's a lifestyle plan.

It's something that you'll easily be able to do for a very long time to come. This is great news when compared to other nutrition plans. Every day when you wake up, you think to yourself, "Dang another day of boring eating, I'm not sure how much longer I can handle this." And most people don't last long on boring diet plans that have them eating the same bland foods day in and day out.

With that being said, you'll of course want to limit certain food choices on the DASH diet. You can certainly include these things as part of your 5 servings of sweets per week, but be cautious not to overdo it. The servings and calories can add up rather quickly if you do! This list isn't meant to scare you into not eating any of these foods, but rather to help you better understand why they need to be limited in order for you to be successful with the DASH diet plan.

Processed foods:

Processed foods are made with certain ingredients that will extend the shelf life of those foods. On one hand, this seems great. It allows the expiration date of a food item to be extended longer so we can take a longer time to eat the food if we wish.

However, we have to take a step back and consider the harmful effects these ingredients can have on our bodies over the long haul. Here are some reasons why you'll want to limit the consumption of processed foods:

Empty calories: processed foods in most cases contain a lot of empty calories. Imagine eating broccoli for example. This vegetable is rich in a lot of key vitamins and nutrients that your body needs. It doesn't contain a lot of calories, and the calories that it does contain are jam-packed with healthy nutrients.

On the flip side, consider a processed food item such as a candy bar. The candy bar doesn't contain very many beneficial vitamins and minerals for our bodies. It also contains a lot of calories from simple sugars. That's why the calories from something like a candy bar are considered to be empty. They're providing your body with nothing useful that it needs.

So you'll likely be unable to get full and stay satisfied, meaning that you'll have to eat even more calories. This is why you must be cautious when eating processed foods. The calories won't do much to keep you full, and it can be very easy to overeat them.

High in trans fat and processed oils: Remember that on the DASH diet we are seeking to eliminate or greatly limit the amount of trans fat that we're consuming. Most processed foods contain quite a bit of trans fat and processed oils that we'll want to avoid. These kinds of fats are high in Omega-6 fatty acids.

Omega-6 fatty acids by themselves are not bad, however they can become a problem when consumed in excess compared to Omega-3 fatty acids. Omega-6 fatty acids cause our bodies to become inflamed. Excess inflammation can cause damage to our joints, impede recovery, and cause heart disease among other things (14).

This is why it's important to have a balance of Omega-3 fatty acids, which act as an anti-inflammatory in the body. The Omega-3 fatty acids can help to counteract the inflammation from the Omega-6 fatty acids.

Low in fiber: processed foods contain a low amount of fiber. Other foods like fruits and vegetables contain high amounts of fiber. As I've talked about earlier, fiber is not only important for our digestive health, but it's also very important for keeping us full for longer periods of time.

This is the real danger of eating too much processed foods. They don't fill you up very well, so you have to eat more of them to get full. This likely means that you'll eat more calories than you should have.

Contain simple carbohydrates: Some people think that you should avoid carbs at all costs, and it's easy to believe considering how bad of a reputation carbs have been getting lately. However, all of this hate on carbs isn't justified. There are good carbs and bad carbs.

Not all carbs are evil and should be avoided like the plague. There are two different kinds of carbohydrates—simple and complex. Simple carbs are carbs that are quickly broken down and processed by the body. This is a bad thing because the rapid breakdown leads to a spike in your insulin levels.

Insulin spikes can lead to food cravings at random times, and your body doesn't burn fat while your insulin levels are high (15).

Conversely, there are complex carbohydrates. These are carbs such as brown rice and sweet potatoes. These kinds of carbs are slower digesting carbs that will not cause spikes in your blood sugar levels. Complex carbs are considered to be a healthy carb that also contains many beneficial vitamins and nutrients.

Sodas:

Sodas should be severely limited if not completely eliminated on the DASH diet. Limiting or eliminating soda intake is one of the first steps I have people take to start losing weight. The reason is similar to why you'd want to limit your intake of processed foods. Sodas contain an excessive amount of sugar, high fructose corn syrup, and empty calories.

Unlike certain processed foods, I consider soda and candy to be the ultimate forms of empty calories because they literally contain only sugar. They provide absolutely zero nutrition that's beneficial for your body. Soda and candy will do nothing to keep you full, and they'll give you random cravings—not good at all!

Excessive amounts of sugar have been linked to many negative health effects such as increased fat mass, increased amount of triglycerides in the blood, insulin resistance, and increase in low-density lipoproteins (the bad form of cholesterol) among other things (16). So needless to say, soda is something you'll definitely want to watch out for.

The thing is sugar can be quite addicting (17), so how can you start to limit your soda intake if it's currently too high? I would avoid trying to quit cold turkey. Imagine if you've been drinking an average of two sodas per day for the last five years.

Is it really that likely you'll be able to walk away from it and never look back? Doubtful. Instead, you need to take a more steady approach. If for example, you're drinking 16 ounces of soda per day, then start off by pouring out 4 ounces of the soda and diluting the remaining 12 ounces with 4 ounces of water.

After doing that for a week, take another step forward by pouring out 8 ounces of soda and diluting the remaining 8 ounces of soda with 8 ounces of water. From there, once that week has finished, you can do 4 ounces of soda with 12 ounces of water. And then move completely away from it.

Sure it's tempting to want to go all out and eliminate soda completely in one fell swoop, but know yourself and be wise. If you think you'd be more successful by being patient and gradually easing yourself off of soda, then do that.

Juices and other artificially sweetened beverages

Wait what? I thought things like orange juice were good for you? Yes, if you took oranges, squeezed them, and only drank the juice that came directly from the oranges that would be ok.

However, most fruit juices and other artificially sweetened beverages aren't healthy options. The main reason why is because they are loaded with a bunch of excessive sugar. Most juices don't contain purely the sugar found in the fruits.

Most of the time, there's added sugar in the juices. Yes, these juices do contain a lot of vitamins such as vitamin A and C, however this doesn't make them a healthy drink option. In fact, this deceives people into thinking that it's a healthy choice when the truth is that it's not.

If you want to get more vitamin A and C in your diet, then eat more fruits and vegetables. You don't have to go out of your way by drinking more fruit juices to get more vitamins. Yes, it's easier to consume these vitamins by drinking them, but it comes at a cost. And that cost is excessive amounts of sugar.

As mentioned earlier, too much sugar in the diet has been shown to lead to health problems such as metabolic syndrome, certain types of cancer, and diabetes. In addition to that, sugar has been shown to be highly addictive, so you must be careful with how much you consume. It's certainly best to avoid the unnecessary sugar and get your vitamins and nutrients from whole food sources such as fruits and vegetables.

White Bread

On the DASH diet, you're going to consuming whole grains, such as whole-wheat bread. Something you'll want to avoid is white bread. On the surface, it might appear as if bread is bread so what's the big deal with white bread? Why do we want to avoid eating it whenever possible?

For starters, white bread is a simple carbohydrate. As I talked about earlier, simple carbs should be avoided in favor of complex carbs. Simple carbohydrates provide little nutritional value to your body, and they also cause rapid spikes in your blood sugar levels, which can lead to food cravings at random times throughout the day.

Not only that, but white bread ranks high on the glycemic index scale (GI scale for short). The GI scale measures how fast or slow different carbohydrates cause increases in blood glucose levels. The slower the carbohydrate increases blood glucose levels, the better it is, and thus the lower the score it'll receive on the glycemic index scale.

The scale ranges from 0-100, and basically what you need to know is that the closer a food item is to 0, the better it is for you. White bread has a GI score of 75 (18), which isn't good at all. It'll quickly raise blood sugar levels much faster than other carbohydrates will. That's why on the DASH diet, you'll be consuming whole grains, which rank much lower on the glycemic index scale. And you'll want to greatly limit or completely avoid carbs such as white bread.

French Fries

French fries are essentially the fried version of a potato. Now there's nothing wrong with a regular white potato or a sweet potato. However, when you take a potato and fry it, many things happen along the way that makes the food item unhealthy. For instance, when the food is being cooked, it's being fried in unhealthy oils.

This is going to drastically increase the amount of fat content in the food. Not only that but when you order fries from a fast food restaurant, what are they going to add to the fries? That's right, they're going to add salt. This will unnecessarily increase the amount of sodium in the food.

And as you learned from earlier, taking in too much sodium can cause hypertension, which is why you'll want to limit sodium intake on the DASH diet. Finally, fries are very easy to over consume. Think about how long it takes you to eat a potato or sweet potato. Now compare that to how long it takes you to wolf down a side of medium fries from a fast food restaurant.

And since these fries contain a lot of added fat, this means that they contain an excessive amount of calories as well. Plus you won't be eating the fries plain as they are, of course you'll have to dip them in ketchup with contains high fructose corn syrup and more sugar than you'd think. Fries are definitely something you can overeat rather quickly, so be very cautious of this food on the DASH diet.

Cookies, cakes, and other pastries

These sweet treats are another simple carbohydrate that you'll want to watch out for. Their nutritional content is made up primarily of refined sugars and other processed ingredients. These foods usually contain shortening, which is a type of solid fat that's high in saturated fat. This is one of the bad types of fat that you'll want to limit whenever possible. Yes, these foods are tasty, but be wary not to over consume them as part of your 5 servings per week following the nutritional plan.

Chapter 4: Health Benefits of the DASH Diet

Chances are good that you want to start the DASH diet eating plan because you want to improve your health. What health benefits can you expect to gain from following this nutrition plan? Well, quite a few things as it turns out.

The DASH diet has been voted to be the best diet 6 years in a row by U.S. News and World Report (19). Obviously there must be many great things about it to be able to uphold that type of a standard. Let's go ahead and jump into those benefits right now:

Health Benefit #1: Lowering of Cholesterol

Cholesterol is a waxy substance found in most of your body's tissues. It's mostly made in the liver, but cholesterol can also be found in foods such as eggs, butter, and cheese. When most people hear the word cholesterol, they think of something negative and unhealthy, but that actually isn't the case.

Cholesterol is necessary for the building of new cells. It only becomes a problem when the amount of cholesterol in the blood becomes too high. Most people don't realize that there are two different kinds of cholesterol— high-density lipoproteins (HDL's) and low-density lipoproteins (LDL's). Your high-density lipoproteins are your body's good type of cholesterol and it's responsible for carrying your LDL's to the liver to be disposed of, and it stops the build-up of LDL's in the arteries.

As you can probably already guess, low-density lipoproteins are your body's bad type of cholesterol, and LDL's stick to artery walls, narrow artery walls, and cause plaque build-up. In reality, if you're looking to lower your cholesterol levels, what you're actually wanting to do is decrease your bad cholesterol levels (aka your LDL's), and you're looking to increase the amount of good cholesterol (aka your HDL's).

The main way the DASH diet is going to work to lower your bad cholesterol levels is by controlling the foods you eat—specifically your fat intake in this case. When we eat a lot of high fatty foods, this can cause issues with our cholesterol levels if we're not careful. This is especially true if the fat content we're eating is saturated fat and trans fat.

These are unhealthy types of fat that'll be limited on the DASH eating plan. Once these types of fat are severely limited or eliminated completely, you won't be raising your low-density lipoprotein levels, but rather decreasing them. Not all fats will be completely eliminated on the DASH diet of course.

And the healthy fats that you'll be consuming will help to increase the good type of cholesterol in your body. Additionally, losing weight and exercising regularly will also help to increase the number of high-density lipoproteins in your body, which I'll talk more about later.

Health Benefit #2: Lowering Blood Pressure

This is considered to be the biggest benefit of the DASH diet considering that its name stands for dietary approaches to stop hypertension. But what exactly is blood pressure anyway? Why is lowering your blood pressure so important for your overall health and well being?

Your body needs oxygen and energy in order to properly function. Every time your heart beats, it pumps blood, which contains oxygen and other rich nutrients throughout your entire body. Your blood is carried throughout your body via blood vessels. Your blood pushes against the blood vessels. How hard your blood is pushing up against your blood vessels will determine your blood pressure.

The harder the blood pushes against the vessels, the higher your blood pressure will be. If your arteries are partially clogged with plaque, this will cause your body to have to work harder in order to keep pumping blood throughout your system.

This is why lowering your cholesterol levels can also help you to lower your blood pressure at the same time. Eventually, all of this extra stress and strain on your heart and vessels can lead to serious health problems such as a heart attack or stroke. Having hypertension is certainly no laughing matter, but how can you tell if you have high blood pressure in the first place?

The first thing you'll want to do is measure your blood pressure. You can get this measured by visiting your doctor, going to certain pharmacies, or even by buying your own blood pressure monitor at a store or online. The main thing you'll want to be aware of before taking your reading is that you haven't exercised for the past 2-3 hours.

Exercise increases blood flow in the body, and yes it's a very healthy thing to do, but it'll skew the reading not giving you an accurate picture of where your blood pressure actually is. Aside from that, be sure to follow these tips to ensure an accurate reading of your blood pressure:

1. Use a properly sized cuff that fits your arm size. Using an oversized cuff won't allow the machine to properly read your blood pressure, and using an undersized cuff will squeeze too tightly and be uncomfortable.

2. Sit in a chair with your arm resting on an armrest. You want your arm to be in a relaxed position instead of strained when the measurement is being taken.

3. Use an arm cuff whenever possible over a wrist cuff. The arm cuff provides a more accurate measurement of your blood pressure than a wrist cuff does.

4. Stay still and quiet while the measurement is being taken. Talking and moving can mess up the reading.

5. If possible, try to keep your upper arm at the same level as your heart.

6. Place the cuff around the bare skin of your arm and don't inhibit the cuff with any clothing.

Now that you know how to properly take your blood pressure, how do you know if you have high blood pressure or not? You can use the following chart to determine if you have blood pressure in a healthy range:

	Systolic	Diastolic
Normal Blood Pressure	>120	>80
Prehypertension	120-139	80-89
High Stage 1	140-159	90-99
High Stage 2	160+	100+

Note: when you take your blood pressure, you'll see a number like 120/80. The first number (120 in this case) is your systolic blood pressure reading. Your systolic blood pressure is the maximum amount of pressure your heart exerts while beating.

The second number (80 in this example) is your diastolic blood pressure. Your diastolic blood pressure is the measurement of blood pressure in your blood vessels when your heart rests between beats. You would still be considered to have high blood pressure if either reading of your systolic or diastolic blood pressures is high.

Now according to the chart, ideally you want to have a blood pressure reading of less than 120/80. If it's in between the ranges of 120-139/80-89, then you're considered to have elevated blood pressure. You're not considered to have hypertension, but this is something you still need to be cautious of and take the necessary actions to lower it.

If your blood pressure reads between 140-159/90-99, then you're considered to have stage 1 hypertension. If your blood pressure reading measures 160+/100+, then you're considered to have stage 2 hypertension. Stage 2 hypertension is essentially a more serve version of hypertension.

Of course a diagnosis of high blood pressure must be confirmed by a medical professional. If you take a blood pressure reading at home, and you get a high reading, you should see your health care professional for medical guidance and be officially diagnosed with hypertension.

Once you have been officially diagnosed with high blood pressure, what are some things you can do in addition to your doctor's recommendations that can help you lower your blood pressure back down to normal levels?

Tip #1: Stop smoking. If you're currently smoking reducing the amount of cigarettes you smoke or stopping smoking altogether will help you to reduce your blood pressure. The reason for this is because cigarettes contain carbon monoxide. Carbon monoxide decreases your body's ability to carry oxygen, which forces it to have to work harder.

Tip #2: Lose Weight. Carrying around extra weight puts extra strain on your heart. This extra strain in turn forces your heart to have to work harder and thus your blood pressure will increase. The DASH diet will help you to be able to lose weight, which in your will help to decrease your blood pressure.

Tip #3: Limit Alcohol Intake. Drinking excessive amounts of alcohol will increase cortisol levels. Cortisol is a steroid hormone that helps to regulate metabolism and immune response in the body. Research has shown that increased cortisol levels can increase blood pressure (20).

Therefore, by limiting your alcohol intake, you can help to limit unhealthy amounts of cortisol in the body, and thus lower blood pressure. For females, this would mean no more than one alcoholic beverage per day. For males, this would mean no more than 2 alcoholic beverages per day.

And no you can't save it all up and drink it all during the weekend—that's binge drinking! You're still only allowed to have 1-2 drinks per day even on the weekends while on the DASH diet.

Tip #4: Decrease Stress. This may not be the easiest thing to do, but lowering your stress levels can help to decrease your blood pressure. When we are stressed our bodies enter into fight or flight mode. In this state, certain hormones such as adrenaline and cortisol are released to help your body prepare to fight.

Unhealthy amounts of these hormones can increase blood pressure levels. If you're experiencing a lot of stress right now, do what you can to help decrease your stress levels. Practice deep breathing when you notice yourself feeling stressed. Meditate or go for a walk outside. Doing these types of things can help to decrease the amount of stress in your life.

Tip #5: Exercise Regularly. Exercise is a great way to decrease your blood pressure. When you exercise, your blood vessels open up, which allows for more blood flow, and this means that your heart won't have to work as hard thus lowering blood pressure.

Tip #6: Take your medications as prescribed. This tip should be obvious, but it's important to be reminded. Whatever medications you're currently taking, be sure to take them as your doctor has prescribed them to you. Taking the wrong amount of your medications can negatively affect your blood pressure.

Of course following the DASH diet will greatly help you be able to decrease your blood pressure, but these are some additional things you can do to help fight against hypertension.

Health Benefit #3: Weight Loss

Another benefit of the DASH diet (and one I'm sure you're really interested in) is weight loss. Yes, the DASH diet is a great way to help you get back to a healthy bodyweight. The only way your body loses weight is by being in a caloric deficit. A caloric deficit is when your body burns off more calories than you consume.

I'll be going into more specifics about this later on, but for now know that getting in a caloric deficit is critical if you want to lose weight. The DASH diet is a great way to help your body be in a caloric deficit because you're going to be consuming healthier foods such as fruits and vegetables. These types of foods are very nutrient dense, meaning that they contain a lot of vitamins and minerals even though they don't contain a lot of calories.

This is amazing because your body needs certain nutrients in order to feel full and satisfied, which means you'll be able to get full on fewer calories. Imagine when you eat chocolate for example. You can eat a lot of chocolate (which contains a lot of calories) and still not feel full at all.

That won't be the case with the foods you're going to be eating on the DASH diet. Additionally, you'll also be cutting back or completely eliminating certain foods from your diet. Your sugar intake will decrease drastically because you'll only be eating 5 servings of sweets per week. And sugar provides very little if any nutritional value to your body.

You'll also be reducing bad fats such as saturated and trans fat. This'll also help to lower your overall caloric intake because fat contains 9 calories per gram, whereas carbs and protein only contain 4 calories per gram. Even though the DASH diet will be able to help you lose weight, you still must have patience.

The DASH diet isn't like your typical diet fad where you drink a magical formula before bed and lose 10 pounds overnight. No instead, the weight might come off slower than you'd like for it to. You might only lose .5-1 pound per week, but remember this is going to be permanent weight loss. You won't have to worry about gaining this weight back ever again.

Think about how someone gains weight. They usually gain weight slowly and steadily over the years, and then they suddenly realize how much things have gotten out of control. You likely didn't gain all of this weight in a short period of time, so be patient and don't try to lose it all in a short period of time. Remember slow and steady wins the race!

Health Benefit #4: Lower risk of stroke, heart attack, kidney stones, diabetes, and certain types of cancer

When you follow the DASH diet for a long period of time, your chances of developing certain types of diseases is lowered (21). This is great news because health diseases are a big problem in the world right now. Cardiovascular disease is the number one killer in the United States killing over 600,000 Americans each and every year (22).

That's definitely a scary statistic, but there are certainly things within your control that you can do to help lower the risk of developing these diseases. By following the DASH diet, you'll essentially be killing a lot of birds with one stone. The research is sound in showing that when people follow the DASH diet for a significant length of time, their risk for diabetes, certain types of cancer, stroke, and heart attack drops quite a bit (23)(24)(25).

Chapter 5: How to Easily Follow the DASH Diet for a Long Time to Come

When most people start a diet are they successful with it? Sadly no, most people who start a diet, aren't able to stick with it for a very long time, and they're not able to get any noticeable results because of it. If you've ever tried a diet in the past and failed, don't worry, it's not your fault. In most cases, the diet sets you up to fail right from the start.

Luckily the DASH diet isn't like your average diet. It's smart in it's approach to helping you lose weight and get in better health. It's designed in a way to help you be able to sustain the diet for a long time to come. However, even with that being the case, there are some extra things you can do ensure long-term success with the DASH diet eating plan. The following are some good tips and tricks you can use to make sure you get long-term results with this nutrition plan:

Tip #1: Don't Beat Yourself Up

One of the worst things you can do on the DASH diet (or any diet for that matter) is to beat yourself up or feel incredibly guilty whenever you slip up. We're all humans, which means that we're not perfect and we'll make mistakes from time to time. For example, you might eat more ice cream, cake, or another sweet treat than you should of.

What do most people do when they slip up on their diets? They start to feel incredibly guilty, and then since they feel as if their diet is already ruined, they might as well go ahead and eat how they please. This will then of course ruin their nutrition plan indefinitely. Conversely, you must be different from the average person by expecting mistakes to occur when you start the DASH diet plan.

Think about it—if you're going to follow this diet plan for years and years to come, is it really realistic to expect that you'll do everything perfectly and never mess up? Of course it's not! That's why you'll want to set realistic expectations going into the diet.

When you do mess up, take a deep breath and stay calm. Tell yourself it's ok and things like this will happen from time to time. Whenever you fall off track, you can always get back up and keep going. Most people however, feel so ashamed that they decide to give up completely. The only way you will not succeed is if you quit. If you persist and keep going, you'll succeed. Sure there will be some bumps in the road, and it won't be the easiest thing you've ever done, but that's the point!

Anything worth achieving is going to be difficult to achieve. Yes, it might be hard to lose weight and get your blood pressure in check, but the reward will be well worth it. So by planning for and expecting things to not go smoothly 100% of the time, you'll be much more prepared for how you'll need to handle these hic-ups.

Tip #2: Have the Right Mindset Going Into the DASH Diet

Yes the DASH eating plan is technically a "diet," and that's how I've mentioned it throughout this book, but I don't like referring to the DASH eating plan as a diet. When you think of a diet, what do you usually think of? To me when I hear someone say, "I'm going on a diet," I think of something you'll do for the short-term.

You'll go *on* a diet, which means that you'll eventually have to go *off* that same diet. I think of someone who's tired of his or her current health or the way that they look in the mirror. They'll do anything to get some results as quickly as possible. So they'll jump right into an unrealistic diet where they cut out all of the junk food in their diet. Sure they'll get some results at first, but when they can't take it anymore, they'll quit and gain all of the weight back.

And that's the biggest problem with diets. They don't imply long-term, permanent change. They imply putting yourself through a bunch of misery for as long as you can. Then when you can't take it anymore, you give up, and you go back to the way you were eating before you started the diet.

The DASH diet really isn't as much of a diet as it is a lifestyle change. This is how you need to think about the DASH nutrition plan heading into it. If you think about it in terms of a lifestyle change instead of a diet, you'll be much more successful with it. When you think about someone making a lifestyle change, what comes to mind? Probably something positive like lasting changes and thus lasting results.

Now of course does this mean you could take any regular diet, call it a lifestyle change, and poof it's easier to do and you'll be successful with it? No of course not! If a diet is unrealistic from the start, there's no way you'll be able to stick with it for a long time to come. Simply eating nothing but healthy foods such as fruits and vegetables and calling that a lifestyle change instead of a diet is going to have little impact on your results.

The difference with the DASH plan is that it's set up in a way that allows you to actually execute it as a lifestyle change. This is because it allows you to eat up to 5 servings per week of sweets. Doing something like completely eliminating all sweets from your nutrition plan is unrealistic, which is why you'd have to refer to it as a diet.

That's not the case with the DASH eating plan. You're set up from the start to be able to do it for a long time to come, which is far better than most eating plans that fail you before you've even begun.

Tip #3: Actually Eat Your 5 Servings of Sweets per Week

Remember what I just mentioned in the previous step—the DASH plan can be done for a long time to come because it allows you to enjoy your favorite foods from time to time. Even with this being the case, it can still be tempting to want to skip the sweets in an effort to try and obtain even faster results.

I'm telling you right now that you need to avoid that temptation. Eating the sweets (or whatever else you like) is a big part of the eating plan. It'll help to restore your leptin levels, which is an important hormone that regulates how much we eat by telling the brain the amount of fat that's stored in our bodies fat cells.

When we eat sweet treats (such as cake for example) that increases the amount of leptin in our bodies, and this increased leptin will allow us to burn more fat. If we're solely eating low amounts of calories from healthy foods, then our leptin stores will be low, and this will signal to our brains that we need to eat more and hold onto the fat that we currently have stored up.

Not only that, but it's going to give you a break and allow you to reward yourself for eating healthy the rest of the time. Think about it, most people work 5 days and then they have 2 days off, which allows them to relax, recover, and prepare themselves for the following workweek. Imagine if you never got a single day off in your life!

That's essentially what it would be like if you never ate another sweet again in your life. Since this is a lifestyle change, you must be patient. The results will eventually come, and once they do come, you won't have to worry about them going away.

People start to do unrealistic things that won't last when they want fast results. Ironically enough, these people end up achieving no results over a long period of time all because they were chasing something that wasn't going to work from the get-go. Be patient and follow the eating plan exactly as you're supposed to, and you'll have nothing to worry about. And yes that does include eating the 5 servings of sweets per week!

Chapter 6: What Kind of Exercise Works Best with the DASH Diet?

Yes, the DASH diet is a great nutritional plan by itself, but there's another important element we can't forget about—exercise. Of course the DASH diet by itself will certainly be able to provide you with many great health benefits, but these benefits can be maximized with the addition of exercise. The research is clear when it comes to exercise (26). It'll provide the following benefits to you:

- Reduce your risk of cardiovascular disease, stroke, and diabetes
- Make you feel happier
- Reduce feelings of anxiety, depression, and stress
- Help you lose weight
- Help prevent osteoporosis
- Build muscle
- Improve brain health
- Improve sleep quality
- Help you relax
- Increase energy

Yes, you'll notice that many of these benefits of exercise are similar to the pros of the DASH diet. This doesn't mean that you shouldn't exercise because you'll already experience these benefits with your nutrition plan. Instead, this should make you want to exercise more because exercising will amplify these amazing health benefits.

Instead of simply reducing your risk of heart attack and stroke, why not make the risk as low as possible by combining the powers of nutrition with exercise? I get it—most of us are busy people. We have school, work, and a family we have to take care of.

But lack of time is no good excuse for not exercising more. This myth of not having time to workout came about because people think that they have to workout for a long time in order for it to be effective. And you're right, if you had to be in the gym for hours a day, then it'd be reasonable to think that you don't have enough time to workout.

But that isn't the case—you can start to experience some of the benefits of exercise (such as improvement of mood and energizing your body) just by taking a brisk walk for 10 minutes. That equates to less than 1% of your day!

What Type of Exercise Should You Do?

Now that you know the importance of exercise, the real question is what kind of exercise you should be doing. Of course there are many different things that you could be doing and none of them are bad. However, I do think that different things work best for different kinds of people.

At the end of the day, the best kind of exercise for you is the kind of exercise you'll actually do. You might like cardio more than weightlifting or vice-versa and that's ok. Ideally you would do both because there are certain benefits you can only get from doing cardio, and there are certain benefits you can get from weightlifting. With that being said, let's get into some specifics for what you should be doing in terms of exercise:

Weightlifting

Many times when people think of lifting weights, they think of macho bodybuilders. You don't have to have the end goal of looking like a bodybuilder if you want to lift weights. And no, lifting weights won't make you look like a bodybuilder. Resistance training has been shown to increase bone density, which can help to prevent osteoporosis when you're older (27).

Weightlifting is also great for building and maintaining muscle mass. You may or may not be interested in building muscle mass, but it'll decrease as you age. This decrease in muscle mass can lead to disability and injury. The cool thing is that you don't have to workout 5-6 times a week to start seeing these benefits.

Studies have shown that you only need to engage in resistance training 2-3 times per week to start reaping the rewards (28). Of course, you may not be sure what to do when you're at the gym but fear not. The following is a good workout you can do as a beginner to lifting weights:

- Back Squats 3 sets of 10 reps 90 seconds rest between sets
- Dumbbell Military Press 3 sets of 10 reps 60 seconds rest between sets
- Lat Pulldown 3 sets of 12 reps 60 seconds rest between sets
- Incline Dumbbell Bench Press 3 sets of 8 reps 90 seconds rest between sets
- Standing Dumbbell Curls 3 sets of 10 reps 60 seconds rest between sets
- Tricep Rope Pushdowns 3 sets of 12 reps 60 seconds rest between sets
- Planks 3 sets of holding the plank position for as long as you can

Side Note #1: A set is a group of consecutive repetitions. A repetition is one complete motion of an exercise. And the rest period is how long of a break you'll take until you start the next set.

For example, let's say you're completing 3 sets of 10 reps and resting 90 seconds in between sets for the barbell squat exercise. You'll squat down and stand back up, completing the movement of the exercise and one rep. You'll repeat that motion 9 more times for a total of 10 repetitions. That will complete the set and you will begin your rest period.

Once your 90-second rest period is up, you'll start the next set and perform another 10 repetitions. That will complete set number 2, and you'll rest another 90 seconds. Once that time period is up, you'll complete the final set of 10 repetitions, and then you'll move onto the next exercise.

Side Note #2: Lift as much weight as you possibly can for the given rep range. Initially, you won't know how much weight to use so you'll have to take your best guess. For example, let's say you're doing bench press for 8 reps. You think you can lift around 150 pounds for that many reps, but on your first set, you easily complete 10 reps.

This means the weight is too light and you need to increase it for the next set. On the next set, you lift 165 pounds and struggle to complete the 8th rep. This is what you want to happen and it means you've found a good weight to use. Once you can complete all 3 sets of 8 reps with 165 pounds, move up to 170 the next time you bench press. If you can't complete 8 reps for all 3 sets, stick with 165 until you can. Here's an example:

Workout 1: Bench Press with 165 pounds
Set 1: 8 reps
Set 2: 8 reps
Set 3: 7 reps

Because you only completed 7 reps on the last set, stick with 165 for the next workout—

Workout 2: Bench Press with 165 pounds

Set 1: 8 reps
Set 2: 8 reps
Set 3: 8 reps

Because you completed all 3 sets of 8 reps, move up to 170 on your next workout with bench press.

It's better to use a weight that's too heavy and miss a rep or two than it is to use a weight that's too light and leave some reps in the tank. For example, it's better to do 170 pounds and only complete 6 reps instead of 8 opposed to using 155 pounds and stopping at 8 reps even though you could've easily done more reps.

Side Note #3: You can set up your gym schedule however you like based on the number of days you're going to be working out. The specific days of the week you workout versus when you rest isn't important.

For example, if you're going to workout 2 times per week you could workout on Tuesday and Friday or Wednesday and Saturday for example. The main thing you'll want to do when working out 2 days per week is have at least 48 hours of rest in between the workouts.

If you're going to workout 3 times per week you could workout on Monday, Wednesday, and Friday. You could also workout on Tuesday, Thursday, and Saturday. Choose whatever works best for you and your schedule. The main thing when you're working out three days per week is to make sure that you're taking at least one day of rest in between your workouts.

Playing Sports

If the idea of running on a treadmill sounds boring to you, then doing something such as playing sports can be a good option for you. Sports are essentially an intense form of cardio disguised in the form of a game.

It doesn't matter what makes you do cardio as long as you do it, and sports are a great way to break up the monotony of doing cardio on a machine. Interestingly enough, playing high-impact sports such as basketball or soccer have been shown to increase bone density more so than non-impact sports such as swimming (29).

Running

Aside from playing sports, you can also go the more traditional route of cardio and do regular running such as jogging or sprinting. You can do long steady-state cardio where you run at the same pace for a certain length of time, or you can do a more intense version of cardio such as high-intensity interval training.

Either form of cardio will provide you with positive health effects. Doing steady-state cardio is simple and doesn't need much explaining—you run at the same pace for a predetermined length of time or distance.

High-intensity interval training (HIIT for short) can be a little bit harder to grasp if you've never heard of it before. HIIT is simply alternating between high-intensity cardio and low intensity cardio. It can be performed by running outside, or on any cardio machine of your choosing at the gym. Here's an example of a HIIT workout you could do on a treadmill:

-Run at 7.5 mph for 1 minute
-Walk at 3.5 mph for 1 minute

Now of course if you need to adjust the intensity of the HIIT then you can certainly do so. You can alter the run-walk ratios (i.e. run for 30 seconds and walk for 1.5 minutes), or you can decrease the intensity of each run (i.e. run at 6 mph instead of 7.5). And if what I prescribed is too easy, then ramp up the intensity accordingly.

Walking

Walking tends to get a bad reputation. People think that it's only something unfit people do. I used to fall into this line of thinking as well and it couldn't be any further from the truth. In fact, there are certain health benefits that you'll get from walking that you can't get from the more intense forms of cardio. For starters, walking is a low-impact form of exercise.

This means that it won't be as strenuous on your bones, tendons, and ligaments as other forms of exercise might be. It's also incredibly simple to do. You don't have to worry about changing into gym clothes and driving to the gym if you don't want to. You can walk just about anywhere whenever you feel like it.

Finally walking helps to cleanse the lymphatic system. While the circulatory system relies on the heart to move blood, the lymphatic system doesn't have a pump like the heart does to keep it going. It instead relies on bodily movement to keep on going.

The lymphatic system is important for ridding the body of toxins, waste, and other unwanted materials. And engaging the lymphatic system is simple; all it really takes is 10-20 minutes of brisk walking per day. This'll be a great start to get the lymphatic system moving and start clearing your body of harmful toxins.

Chapter 7: Setting Up and Starting Your DASH Diet Plan

So far, you've learned a lot of information about the DASH eating plan and what it can do for you. However, putting all of the info together into an actionable plan can be a little confusing and difficult.

In this chapter, I'm going to give you the step-by-step process to set-up your DASH diet nutrition plan so that you can get started with it as soon as possible. Let's dive right in...

Step #1: Don't Forget About Calorie Quantity!

When it comes to calories, many people only regard the quality of the calories as important. For example, an avocado would be considered healthier and therefore better than a candy bar. Yes, the avocado will provide your body with way more vitamins and nutrients than the candy bar ever will. However, depending on the amounts, the avocado will likely contain more calories overall than the candy bar.

This is why you must also take into consideration the quantity of the foods you're eating as well. Many people don't think that it's possible to overeat healthy foods, but it certainly is possible. For example, you could eat the following meal for breakfast:

- 1 cup of oatmeal (300 calories)
- 1 cup of 1% milk (103 calories)

- Handful of blueberries (30 calories)
- 1 tbsp. of almond butter (100 calories)
- 1 slice of toast (75 calories)
- Total calories: 608

608 total calories is quite a lot. Of course, this meal would be very filling and nutritious, but it's still more than most would expect when added up. This is important to know because it's a myth that simply starting a healthy diet, such as the DASH diet, will guarantee weight loss when, in fact, it doesn't.

You must be able to track your calories and understand how your body works in regards to weight loss and weight gain, and it all comes down to energy balance. Every day your body needs the energy to breathe, digest food, regulate body temperature, allow your organs to function, etc. We give our body the energy it needs to perform these functions through the foods that we eat also known as calories.

When we eat more calories than our bodies need (caloric surplus), we'll store some of the calories as fat so we can use them later. When we eat exactly the amount of calories our body needs (maintenance), we'll neither gain nor lose weight. And finally, when we eat fewer calories than our body needs (caloric deficit), we'll use some of our stored fat for energy. Here's an example:

Let's pretend that Craig's maintenance calories are 2,300 (don't worry, we'll figure this out in the next step).

- If Craig eats more than 2,300 calories, he'll be in a caloric surplus and will start to gain weight.
- If Craig eats right at 2,300 calories, he'll be eating at his maintenance levels and will neither gain nor lose weight.
- If Craig eats less than 2,300 calories, he'll be in a caloric deficit and will start losing weight.

So if Craig wants to start losing weight, he knows he must eat less than 2,300 calories per day. That's a great start that most people will never even consider. The next thing he must determine is what he eats because it does matter. The point isn't to eat whatever you want as long as you're in a deficit. The point is to plan ahead so you know the direction you're heading in and to eat high-quality foods to feel great and get healthy.

For example, let's say you eat 150 calories worth of fruit and vegetables, and I eat 150 calories from a chocolate bar. Are we equal? Well kinda. The total amount of calories we ate was the same.

There's no arguing this because a calorie *is* a calorie, just like a yard of wood is the same length as a yard of sheet metal. However, the quality of the calories is vastly different. The fruits and vegetables you ate will provide you with fiber, keeping you fuller for a longer period of time. The fruits and vegetables also contain way more vitamins and minerals than the chocolate bar does.

And when you're eating fewer calories overall to lose weight, it's important that you make those calories count. You want to be consuming high-quality foods because that's how you'll stay full for long periods of time even when your calories are being restricted. Now let's move on and determine how many calories you should be eating...

Step #2: Determine Your Resting Metabolic Rate

Like I mentioned in the previous step, your body needs energy (calories) in order to continue on with all of its chemical functions like breathing, digesting food, organ function, etc. The amount of calories you burn on any given day is your resting metabolic rate (rmr). Once you figure out your body's rmr, you can then determine how many calories you need to eat to start burning fat.

Determining your rmr is simple—multiply your bodyweight in pounds by 13.
Let's use myself as an example:

Bodyweight=205 pounds
205 x 13= RMR of 2,665

This means that if I eat less than 2,665 calories, I'll be in a caloric deficit and will start to lose weight. If I eat more than 2,665 calories, I'll be in a caloric surplus and will start to gain weight. And finally, if I eat exactly 2,665 calories, I'll be at maintenance and will neither gain nor lose weight.

The question is—how big of a caloric deficit do you need to create in order for it to translate into pounds lost? There are about 3,500 calories in one pound of fat (30), meaning that you must create a cumulative caloric deficit of 3,500 calories in order to lose 1 pound. So if you divide 3,500 by 7 days in a week, you'll need to create an average daily caloric deficit of 500 calories to lose 1 pound per week.

Referring back to the example from above, here's what that would translate to:

RMR- 2,665 − 500= 2,165

This means that I need to eat 2,165 calories every day if I want to lose 1 pound per week. The more weight you have to lose, the larger the caloric deficit you can create. For example, you could eat at a caloric deficit of 750 calories and lose 1.5 pounds per week, or you could eat at a deficit of 1,000 calories to lose 2 pounds per week.

Essentially, for every 250 calories you can expect to lose an additional .5-pound. The key is to not get carried away. You might want to lose all of the weight as soon as possible and jump right into a 1,000-calorie caloric deficit.

That may not be the best idea. For most people, losing 1 pound per week by creating a 500-calorie caloric deficit is golden. Imagine yourself a year from now being 52 pounds lighter without having to put forth much effort! That's much better than spinning your wheels trying to lose 100 pounds in that same time frame.

Of course you may not be doing the DASH diet to lose weight, and it's okay if that's the case for you. If you're following the DASH eating plan to get some of the health benefits out of it, then you certainly don't have to be nearly as strict in regards to how many calories you're eating.

You'll still want to eat the right foods of course, but you won't have to be as strict with keeping track of your calories. Of course you still can if you want to, just to make sure you stay on track with maintaining your bodyweight. For example, let's say you determined your resting metabolic rate was 2,000 calories. You could still measure out and eat 2,000 calories a day to ensure that you won't gain any unwanted weight.

Step #3: Determine Serving Sizes

Now that you know how many calories it is that you need to be eating, all you need to do from here is start eating according to the DASH diet plan. In an earlier chapter, I went over the number of servings you need to eat per day for each food group. Before I get into how to adjust serving sizes based on your caloric needs, how can you tell how much a serving size is?

Serving sizes will vary depending on the type of food that you're eating. For example, one serving of raw broccoli is ½ cup. On the other hand, 1 cup of milk is a serving of dairy. Unfortunately, it's not as easy as saying one cup of anything equals one serving size.

The best thing you can do is read the nutritional label of the foods you're eating to see what the measured serving sizes are. Sometimes you'll have to eyeball the amount of food you're eating and that's okay. Here's a chart to give you some accurate measurements when you have to eyeball the amount of food you're eating:

Item	Approximate Equivalency
Baseball	~1 cup
Small Computer Mouse	~1/2 cup
Deck of Cards	~3 ounces of meat
Golf Ball	~1 ounce/2 tbsp.
CD	~1 ounce of sliced meat
Nine-Volt Battery	~1 ounce of cheese

In addition to using the eyeball test, you can also buy a food scale. A food scale will be able to tell you how many grams are in a certain food item, which you can then use to determine the serving size. Now, in the earlier chapter, the following serving sizes were recommended for each of these different food groups:

- Vegetables: 4-5 servings per day
- Fruit: 4-5 servings per day
- Nuts, Seeds, and Dried Beans: 3 servings per week
- Dairy: 2-3 servings per day
- Meats, Poultry, and Fish: 1-2 servings per day
- Fats and Oils: 2 per day
- Whole Grains: 6-8 per day
- Sweets: 5 per week

These recommendations are based on a standard 2,000 calorie a day diet. In fact, everywhere you look, food labels and percentages are based on a 2,000 calorie a day diet. The reason why it was set up this way was to because the FDA needed benchmarks for average calorie consumption and 2,000 was the number they came up with.

They knew that people have varying caloric needs, but putting different daily percentage values for a wide range of caloric intakes would take up way too much space. 2,000 is also a very easy number to work with if you need to convert certain values to meet your needs.

So if from the previous steps, you determined that you need to eat 1,600 calories per day, does this mean that you should eat the serving size recommendations for a 2,000 calorie diet? Definitely not! You'll want to make sure that you adjust the serving sizes accordingly to fit your specific needs. Here are a couple of different charts you can use to help you determine your serving sizes based on your caloric needs.

Serving Sizes based on a 1,600 calorie per day diet:

- Vegetables: 3-4 per day
- Fruits: 3-4 per day
- Nuts, Seeds, and Dried Beans: 2 per week
- Dairy: 2 per day
- Meats, Poultry, and Fish: 1 per day
- Fats and Oils: 1-2 per day
- Whole Grains: 6 per day
- Sweets: 3-4 per week

Serving Sizes based on a 3,000 calorie per day diet:

- Vegetables: 6 per day
- Fruits: 6 per day
- Nuts, Seeds, and Dried Beans: 1 per day
- Dairy: 3-4 per day
- Meats, Poultry, and Fish: 2-3 per day
- Fats and Oils: 3-4 per day
- Whole Grains: 10-12 per day
- Sweets: 6-7 per week

These charts will help to cover a wider range of caloric needs, but what if you need to eat 1,800 calories per day for example? In that case, go in between the 2,000 and 1,600 calorie per day plan to figure out approximately how many servings you need to be eating per day.

For example, on the 1,600 calorie plan, you'll be eating 6 servings of whole grains per day. On the 2,000 calorie diet plan, you'll be eating 6-8 servings of whole grains per day. Therefore, if you needed to eat 1,800 calories per day, you could eat 7 servings of whole grains per day.

The 1,600 calorie plan also calls for 3-4 servings of vegetables per day, and the 2,000 calorie diet plan calls for 4-5 servings of vegetables per day. If you're eating 1,800 calories per day, you should therefore eat 4 servings of vegetables per day.

The main goal with servings isn't to get it down exactly right, but to give you a good estimate of how much you should be eating of certain food groups. If you're eating 1,800 calories per day, and you eat 5 servings of vegetables one day, don't sweat it. The main point is to give you an estimation of how you should be eating.

Step #4: Execute on the DASH Eating Plan

Congratulations, by this point you've completed most of the hard work in setting up your nutrition plan! All you need to do is follow through. You know how many calories it is that you should be eating per day, and you also know how much of each food group you should be eating.

All you have to do from here is execute and start getting results! Of course, this isn't the last step in the process because things don't always go exactly the way they're planned out. Sometimes we have to make adjustments along the way...

Step #5: Make Necessary Adjustments

In order to know that you're getting all of the numbers to line up accordingly, you'll need to track how many calories it is that you're eating. Remember, what gets measured gets managed. The best way to be able to do this is to download a calorie counting app on your smartphone. All you have to do is type in the foods that you ate, and in what amounts, and the app will track the how many calories you've eaten for the day.

This is an extremely easy way to make sure that you're on track to hit your caloric goals as well as your serving sizes for the different food groups. Of course, you don't have to use a calorie counting app if you don't want to. You can use a pen and paper if you're old school. It might be a little bit more tedious, but it's still effective.

Simply measure out how many calories are in the foods you're eating by looking at the food label or weighing it on a food scale. From there, you'll simply write down what foods you ate and the total number of calories it contained. Then at the end of the day, you can add up your totals to see where you stand.

Yes, calorie counting is tedious, but there's no other way you're going to be able to fully know if you're on the right track or not. By measuring your calories, you'll be able to know exactly where you stand, and you'll be able to make any necessary adjustments. For example, let's say you need to eat 2,000 calories a day on the DASH diet.

Unless you track what you're eating, how do you really know that you're eating 2,000 calories a day? You simply don't! Once you start tracking your calories, you might realize that you've been eating 2,300 calories per day instead of 2,000—whoops!

That's why it's critical that you measure and track how much food it is that you're eating. After a while, you'll get a good feel for how much it is that you need to eat per day. At that point, you can start to eyeball things more and be less strict with measuring your calories. Until you reach that point though, track your calories!

Ultimately, the point of all of these steps is to teach you how to be self-sufficient with the DASH diet plan. Remember the old saying, if you give a man a fish, you feed him for a day. If you teach a man how to fish, you feed him for a lifetime. Sure I could simply tell you to eat these certain foods and start getting results, but I know that won't last.

In order to get lasting results, you need to be adaptable and make certain adjustments when necessary. Your caloric needs won't always stay the same for example, or you might need to change up serving size for a certain food group. If I simply told you what to do and then ran away, you'd be left clueless as to what to do. Instead my goal is to not just give you the necessary tools you need to be successful with the DASH diet, but also teach you how to use those tools.

That's why following this last step of the process is so important. If you don't measure your weight, you won't know how many calories you need to eat. If you don't know how many calories you need to eat, then you won't know the proper serving sizes for each food group.

And finally, if you don't measure and track what you're eating, then you won't know if you're eating the proper amounts of each food group. It all comes down to preparation. When you fail to prepare, you prepare to fail!

Chapter 8: 14-Day DASH Diet Sample Meal Plan

The following is a 14-day sample meal plan you can use to give you an idea of how you should be eating while on the DASH diet plan. This is simply meant to help guide you and ease you into starting the nutrition plan. It's not to be used as a crutch.

Recall the phrase, "if you give a man a fish, you feed him for a day. If you teach a man to fish, you feed him for life." It wouldn't be practical for me to tell you exactly how to eat each and every day. If I tried to do that, you would end up failing.

You wouldn't be able to adapt to different situations you'd find yourself in. For example, let's say you're at an office party, and you're not able to eat exactly what the meal plan laid out for you. What do you do? You'd likely freeze up and paralyze yourself because you don't know how to adapt yourself to the given situation.

On the other hand, if you know all of the ins and outs of the DASH diet (which you should by now), then you'll know what you are and aren't allowed to eat at the office party. You'll still be able to enjoy yourself without having to constantly worry if you broke your diet plan or not. With that being said, this sample meal plan is based on a 2,000 calorie a day diet. Be sure to adjust the serving and portion sizes accordingly to fit your caloric needs.

Note: You can break up these meal plan ideas into smaller meals with snacks if you like. I made the meal plans with just breakfast, lunch, and dinner, but you can modify it to have snacks if that's how you like to eat.

For example, let's say for breakfast you're going to eat 1 cup of oatmeal, 1 cup of skim milk, ½ cup of raspberries, and 1 medium banana. You could skip out on eating the banana as part of your breakfast and instead eat it a couple of hours later as a snack. It can be done either way because it works out to the same amount of calories in the end. Choose whatever works best for you and how it is that you prefer to eat.

Additionally, replace certain foods as necessary. For example, if a meal calls for ½ cup of blueberries and you like raspberries more, then go ahead and eat ½ cup of raspberries instead of blueberries. Or if you like cauliflower more than carrots, then go ahead and replace the carrots with cauliflower.

Yes, variety is good, but don't feel like you have to eat a certain fruit or vegetable that you hate when you could easily replace it with something else. Do what works best for you and will allow you to stick to this diet for a long time to come.

Finally, I didn't include any of the sweets in the meal plan. Feel free to add in whatever sweets you like throughout the week up to your allotted number of servings.

Day 1:

Breakfast

- 2 Slices of Whole Wheat Toast
- 2 Tablespoons of Natural Peanut Butter (one tbsp. per slice of toast)

- 1 Medium Apple
- ½ Cup of Your Choice of Berries

Lunch

- 3 Ounces of Lean Turkey
- 1 Cup of Broccoli
- 1 Cup of Quinoa
- 1.5 Ounces of Low-Fat Yogurt

Dinner

- 3 ounces of grilled chicken
- ½ Cup of Steamed Cauliflower
- ½ Cup of Steamed Bell Peppers
- 1 Cup of Brown Rice
- 1 Medium Orange

Day 2:

Breakfast:

- 2 Scrambled Eggs
- ½ of a Whole-Wheat Pita Pocket
- ½ of a Medium Grapefruit

Lunch:

- 3 Ounces of Cod
- 2 Teaspoons of Olive Oil
- ½ Cup of Mixed Berries
- 1 Cup of Steamed Broccoli
- 1 Whole-Wheat Roll

Dinner:

- 2 Cups of Whole-Wheat Spaghetti Noodles
- ½ Cup of Grated Parmesan Cheese
- ½ Cup of Tomato Sauce
- 2 Ounces of Lean Beef

Day 3:

Breakfast:

- 1 Cup of Oatmeal
- ½ Cup of Raspberries
- 1 Cup of Skim Milk
- 1 Medium Banana

Lunch:

Salad Consisting of the Following:

- 3 Ounces of Lean Grilled Chicken
- 3 Cups of Leafy Green Vegetables
- ½ Cup of Cumcumber
- ½ Tablespoon of Flax Seeds

On the Side:

- ½ Slice of Toast

Dinner:

- 1 Cup of Roasted Potatoes
- 3 Ounces of Roast Beef
- ½ Cup of Roasted Carrots
- ½ Cup of Roasted Onions

Day 4:

Breakfast:

- 3 Hard Boiled Eggs
- 2 Slices of Turkey Bacon
- 6 Ounces of Freshly Squeezed Orange Juice
- 6 Ounces of Low-Fat Yogurt

Lunch:

Sandwich Consisting of the Following:

- 2 Slices of Whole-Wheat Bread
- 3 Ounces of Packaged Tuna
- 1 Tablespoon of Mayonnaise

On the Side:

- ½ Cup of Kale
- ½ Cup of Tomatoes
- ½ Cup of Spinach
- ½ Cup of Pineapple

Dinner:

- 3 Ounces of Lean Venison
- 1 Cup of Sweet Potatoes
- ½ Cup of Roasted Carrots
- ½ Cup of Roasted Bell Pepper

Day 5:

Breakfast:

Breakfast Sandwich Consisting of the Following:

- 2 Slices of Whole Wheat Toast
- 3 Slices of Turkey Bacon
- 1 Fried Egg

On the side:

- 1 Medium Apple

Lunch:

Turkey Roll-Ups Consisting of:

- 3 Ounces of Lean Turkey Meat
- 1/4 Cup of Cheese
- 2-3 Large Leaves of Romaine Lettuce
- 2 Teaspoons of Mustard

On the Side:

- 1 Medium Apple
- ½ Cup of Mixed Broccoli and Cauliflower

Dinner:

Stuffed Bell Pepper Consisting of:

- 1 Full-Sized Bell Pepper
- 1/4 Cup of Low-Fat Cheese
- ½ Cup of Chickpeas
- ¼ Cup of Dried Apricots

Day 6:

Breakfast:

- 1 Cup of Oat Bran
- 1 Cup of Skim Milk
- ½ Cup of Mixed Berries
- 6 Ounces of Freshly Squeezed Pineapple Juice

Lunch:

Sandwich Consisting of the following:

- 2 Slices of Whole-Wheat Bread
- 3 Ounces of Lean Turkey
- ¼ Cup of Low-Fat Cheese
- 2 Teaspoons of Mustard

On the side:

- 1/3 Cup of Almonds
- 1 Medium Banana
- ½ Cup of Your Choice of Vegetables

Dinner:

Fish Tacos Consisting of:

- 3 Ounces of Tilapia
- 2 Whole-Wheat Tortillas
- 1/4 Cup of Low-Fat Cheese

On the side:

- 1 Medium Peach
- 1 Cup of Mixed Vegetables

Day 7:

Breakfast:

- 1 Whole-Wheat Bagel
- 2 Tablespoons of Natural Almond or Peanut Butter
- 1 Medium Pear
- 1 Cup of Skim Milk

Lunch:

Salad Consisting of the following:

- 4 Cups of Spring Mix Salad
- ¼ Cup of Severed Almonds
- ½ Cup of Orange Slices
- 2 Tablespoons of Low-Fat Dressing

Dinner:

- 3 Ounces of Salmon
- 1 Cup of Strawberries
- 1 Cup of Asparagus
- 1 Small Biscuit
- 2 Teaspoons of Olive Oil

Day 8:

Breakfast:

- 1 Cup of Oatmeal
- 1 Cup of Skim Milk
- ½ Cup of Strawberries
- ½ Cup of Mango

Lunch:

Baked Potato Consisting of the Following:

- 1 Large Potato
- ¼ Cup of Shredded Cheese
- ¼ Cup of Bacon Bits
- 1 Tablespoon of Reduced Fat Sour Cream

On the side:

- 1 cup of mixed broccoli, cauliflower, and bell pepper

Dinner:

- 3 Ounces of Lean Steak
- 1 Cup of Brown Rice
- 1 Teaspoon of Olive Oil
- ½ Cup of Steamed Asparagus and Carrots

Day 9:

Breakfast:

- 2 Slices of Whole-Wheat Toast
- 2 Tablespoons of Natural Almond Butter
- 1 Medium Peach
- 1 Cup of Skim Milk

Lunch:

Salad Consisting of the Following:

- 3 Ounces of Lean Chicken
- 2 Cups of Spring Mix Salad
- 2 Tablespoons of Low-Fat Dressing
- ½ Cup of Raspberries
- 1.5 Ounces of Low-Fat Cheese

Dinner:

Stir Fry Consisting of the Following:

- 2 Cups of Snow Peas
- ½ Cup of Kale
- 2 Tablespoons of Olive Oil
- 2 Cups of Quinoa
- ½ Cup of Mixed Nuts

Day 10:

Breakfast:

- 3 Scrambled Eggs
- 1 Slice of Whole-Wheat Toast
- 2 Slices of Turkey Bacon
- 6 Ounces of Yogurt
- 6 Ounces of Freshly Squeezed Orange Juice

Lunch:

Turkey and Swiss Sandwich Consisting of the Following:

- 3 Ounces of Lean Turkey
- 2 Teaspoons of Mayonnaise
- 2 Slices of a Tomato
- 1 Slice of Swiss Cheese
- 2 Slices of Whole-Wheat Bread

On the side:

½ Cup of Cauliflower and Broccoli

Dinner:

- 2 Cups of Whole-Wheat Angel Pasta
- ½ Cup of Grated Parmesan Cheese
- ½ Cup of Tomato Sauce
- 2 Ounces of Lean Venison
- 1 Cup of Mixed Vegetables

Day 11:

Breakfast:

- 1 Cup of Bran Flakes Cereal
- 1 Cup of Skim Milk
- 1 Medium Apple
- 1 Slice of Whole-Wheat Toast

Lunch:

Turkey Roll-Ups Consisting of:

- 3 Ounces of Lean Turkey Meat
- 1/4 Cup of Cheddar Cheese
- 2-3 Large Leaves of Romaine Lettuce
- 2 Teaspoons of Mustard

On the Side:

- 1 Medium Pear
- ½ Cup of Mixed Brussell Sprouts

Dinner:

Fish Tacos Consisting of:

- 3 Ounces of Cod
- 2 Whole-Wheat Tortillas
- 1/4 Cup of Low-Fat Cheese

On the side:

- ½ of a Medium Grapefruit
- 1 Cup of Mixed Vegetables

Day 12:

Breakfast:

- 1 Cup of Oat Bran
- 1 Cup of Skim Milk
- 1 Medium Orange
- 1 Slice of Whole Wheat Toast
- 1 Tablespoon of Natural Peanut Butter

Lunch:

Salad Consisting of the Following:

- 1 Boiled Egg
- 3 Ounces of Packaged Tuna
- 2 Cups of Leafy Green Vegetables
- ½ Cup of Diced Tomatoes
- 2 Tablespoons of Low-Fat Dressing

Dinner:

Hamburger consisting of the following:

- 3 Ounces of Lean Beef
- 1 Whole-Wheat Bun
- 1 Leaf of Romaine Lettuce
- 1 Slice of a Tomato
- 1 Slice of Cheese
- 2 Teaspoons of Mustard

On the Side:

- 1 Cup of Mixed Vegetables

Day 13:

Breakfast:

Sandwich Consisting of:

- 1 Cooked Egg
- 2 Slices of Turkey Bacon
- 2 Slices of Whole Wheat Toast
- 2 Teaspoons of Mustard
- 1 Slice of Cheese

On the side:

- 1 Medium Banana

Lunch:

Salad Consisting of the following:

- 4 Cups of Spring Mix Salad
- ¼ Cup of Severed Almonds
- ½ Cup of Raspberries
- 2 Tablespoons of Low-Fat Dressing

On the side:

- 1 Whole-Wheat Roll

Dinner:

- 1 Cup of Roasted Sweet Potatoes
- 3 Ounces of Roast Beef
- ½ Cup of Roasted Bell Peppers
- ½ Cup of Roasted Onions

Day 14:

Breakfast:

- 1 Whole-Wheat Bagel
- 2 Tablespoons of Natural Almond or Peanut Butter
- 6 Ounces of Yogurt
- ½ Medium Grapefruit

Lunch:

Sandwich Consisting of:

- 3 Ounces of Lean Chicken Breast
- 2 Slices of Whole Wheat Bread
- 1 Slice of Pepper Jack Cheese
- 1 Slice of a Tomato
- 2 Teaspoons of Mayonnaise

On the Side:

- ½ Cup of Cantaloupe
- ½ Cup of Your Choice of Vegetables

Dinner:

- 3 Ounces of Salmon
- 1 Cup of Brown Rice
- 1 Cup of Cooked Spinach
- 1 Tablespoon of Mixed Nuts
- 1 Whole-Wheat Biscuit

Chapter 9: Frequently Asked Questions

How many meals should I eat per day?

You can eat as many meals as you like throughout the day. Meal frequency doesn't matter for weight loss (31), but the total amount of calories you eat does. So eat however is easiest for you and your schedule.

I myself prefer to eat 3 meals a day and that works great for most people. However, feel free to eat 6 times per day or even as little as once per day. As long as you're hitting your servings for each food group and the correct number of calories you'll be fine.

How Spot On Do I Have to Be With My Serving Sizes?

The serving sizes are there to give you a good idea of how much of certain food groups you should be eating. You don't have to be spot on with each and every food group each and every day—that would drive just about anybody nuts. There might be one day for example where you eat an extra two servings of dairy.

If that's the case, then over the next 2 days you could eat 1 less serving of dairy to balance it out. You're not always going to be perfect with it, and that's ok! What matters is that you stay within a serving or so of what's being recommended and you'll be fine.

How much water should I drink on a daily basis?

Your body is made up of about 60% water, so it's important to consume water for several reasons:

- Helps keep your joints and ligaments fluid, which can help prevent injury
- Helps control your caloric intake
- Flushes out toxins
- Improves skin quality
- Improves kidney function
- Improves your focus

Many people recommend that you should drink 1 gallon of water per day. This is a blanket answer that doesn't meet individual needs. This recommendation would have a 100-pound woman drinking the same amount of water as a 200-pound man. Absurd!

Other health experts advise drinking eight 8-ounce glasses (64 ounces total) of water a day. But again 64 ounces isn't going to be enough for most people. What should you do then? I don't keep track of my water intake—I go by how I feel and the color of my urine.

Your body's own thirst mechanism will be accurate in telling you if you need more water. If you feel thirsty, go drink some water. If not, you're probably ok. You can also use the color of your urine to judge how hydrated you are. If your urine is yellow, then you should drink more water. If it's clear, then you should be good to go. This keeps things simple and it's one less thing you have to keep track of.

How Fast Should I Lose Weight?

The more weight you have to lose, the faster the rate at which you can lose the weight. For example, if you have 50+

pounds to lose, you can lose weight at a rate of 2 pounds or more per week. If you only have 5 pounds to lose, then you'll lose weight at a rate of .5 pound per week.

For most people, losing 1 pound per week is the sweet spot. You'll be creating an average caloric deficit of 500 calories daily. At this pace, you'll be losing weight fairly quickly and you won't be miserable all of the time from a complete lack of calories.

What do I do once I reach my goal bodyweight?

Contrary to what you might be thinking, things aren't going to be that much different from what you've been doing to lose weight. You still need to follow the DASH diet and continue eating in the same manner that you previously were. This means that you should still keep the same eating schedule and keep eating similar meals to the ones that you were eating to lose weight.

However, there's one difference between maintenance and creating a caloric deficit to lose weight. The difference is that you get to consume more calories! How many calories? Well, this is pretty easy to figure out as a matter of fact.

Step #1: Determine at what rate you were losing weight (i.e. 1 pound per week)

Step #2: Translate pounds lost per week into calories
.5-pound lost per week= 250 calories
1 pound lost per week= 500 calories
1.5 pounds lost per week= 750 calories
2 pounds lost per week= 1,000 calories, etc.

Step #3: Add in those additional calories to what you were previously eating to maintain your new weight.

For example, let's say someone was losing weight at a rate of 1 pound per week by eating 1,850 calories per day. Once he hits his goal weight, he needs to eat 2,350 calories (1,850+500) per day to maintain his new weight.

What if I hit a plateau and I stop losing weight at my regular pace?

Let's say you been losing weight just fine, but then all of the sudden you hit a wall and stop losing weight. In this case, take your new current bodyweight (which should be a lower number from when you first started) and multiply that by 13.

Take that number and subtract 250 from it. This will be your new daily caloric intake for you to lose weight.

This will have you losing weight at a rate of approximately .5-pound per week. You may have previously been losing weight at a rate of 1-pound per week, but now you'll lose at a rate of .5-pound per week.

This is because I don't want you to drastically reduce your calories all of the sudden and because if you've hit a plateau you're likely very close to hitting your goal weight anyway.

What if I'm not losing or gaining weight eating 13 calories per pound of bodyweight?

If you've been struggling to lose weight eating 13 calories per pound of bodyweight, then I recommend using a different method to set your calories. Before I get into that though, you must first make sure you were actually eating 13 calories per pound of bodyweight minus 500 calories to lose 1 pound per week. It's easy to overestimate the amount of calories you're eating, and this could be the reason why you're not seeing results.

Once you've made sure you've accurately been tracking your calories, you can take your goal bodyweight, multiply it by 11, and then eat that many calories (don't subtract anything from the final calculated number).

Yes, I understand that your goal bodyweight will be a random number that you think you'll look good at, so take your best guess. Start on the higher side and work your way down from there if you still aren't losing weight.

    Here's an example for a 250-pound male.

        Current Weight 250

        Goal Bodyweight 200

        200x11= 2,200 daily calories

        Let's say once this person reaches his goal of 200 pounds he's still not satisfied with how he looks. From there he can simply set a new goal bodyweight (i.e. 190 pounds for example) and go from there.

Conclusion:

You now know everything about the DASH diet that you need to in order to be successful with it. It's been voted the best diet as many times as it has for good reason. You can certainly get great results with it, and now it's up to you. If you stay dedicated and follow the plan as it is, you'll start to see results. It won't always be easy, but as long as you don't give up, you'll get there in the end! Finally if you have any questions I'd be happy to answer them! You can reach me by emailing me at thomas@rohmerfitness.com Thanks!

Sources

(1) https://www.cdc.gov/bloodpressure/faqs.htm

(2) https://www.cdc.gov/bloodpressure/index.htm

(3) http://www.collective-evolution.com/2017/02/27/shocking-fast-food-statistics-how-you-can-begin-to-eat-better/

(4) https://www.cdc.gov/nchs/fastats/obesity-overweight.htm

(5) https://www.ncbi.nlm.nih.gov/pubmed/15523086

(6) https://www.ncbi.nlm.nih.gov/pubmed/18452640

(7) http://www.nejm.org/doi/10.1056/NEJMoa1501451

(8) https://www.iofbonehealth.org/facts-statistics

(9) https://newsroom.heart.org/news/magnesium-may-modestly-lower-blood-pressure

(10) https://www.ncbi.nlm.nih.gov/pmc/articles/PMC4549665/

(11) https://www.ncbi.nlm.nih.gov/pubmed/27910808

(12) https://www.ncbi.nlm.nih.gov/pmc/articles/PMC3024842/

(13) https://www.ncbi.nlm.nih.gov/pubmed/20329590

(14) https://www.ncbi.nlm.nih.gov/pmc/articles/PMC3335257/

(15) https://www.ncbi.nlm.nih.gov/pubmed/21864752

(16) https://www.ncbi.nlm.nih.gov/pmc/articles/PMC5133084/

(17) https://www.ncbi.nlm.nih.gov/pmc/articles/PMC2235907/

(18) https://www.health.harvard.edu/diseases-and-conditions/glycemic-index-and-glycemic-load-for-100-foods

(19) https://health.usnews.com/best-diet/dash-diet

(20) https://www.ncbi.nlm.nih.gov/pmc/articles/PMC1993964/

(21) https://jamanetwork.com/journals/jamainternalmedicine/fullarticle/414155

(22) https://www.cdc.gov/heartdisease/facts.htm

(23) https://www.ncbi.nlm.nih.gov/pubmed/21058045

(24) https://www.ncbi.nlm.nih.gov/pubmed/26622263

(25) https://www.ncbi.nlm.nih.gov/pubmed/23466047/

(26) https://www.ncbi.nlm.nih.gov/pmc/articles/PMC1402378/

(27) https://www.ncbi.nlm.nih.gov/pubmed/9927006

(28) https://www.ncbi.nlm.nih.gov/pubmed/27102172

(29) https://www.ncbi.nlm.nih.gov/pubmed/11283423

(30) https://www.ncbi.nlm.nih.gov/pmc/articles/PMC2376744/

(31) https://www.ncbi.nlm.nih.gov/pmc/articles/PMC4683169/

Printed in Poland
by Amazon Fulfillment
Poland Sp. z o.o., Wrocław